Liz Hodgkinson has bee
journalist since 1967, sp
in the health field. She h
ing *Smile Therapy, Addict..., ...*
The Alexander Technique. This book brings together her
best-sellers *How to Banish Cellulite Forever* and *The Anti-Cellulite Recipe Book*.

By the same author:

THE ANTI-CELLULITE PLAN

Liz Hodgkinson

Thorsons
An Imprint of HarperCollinsPublishers

Thorsons
An Imprint of HarperCollins*Publishers*
77–85 Fulham Palace Road,
Hammersmith, London W6 8JB
1160 Battery Street,
San Francisco, California 94111-1213

How to Banish Cellulite Forever and
The Anti-Cellulite Recipe Book first
published by Grafton Paperbacks, 1989
and 1990 respectively
First published by Thorsons 1992 and 1990
respectively
This Thorsons edition published 1997

1 3 5 7 9 10 8 6 4 2

A catalogue record for this book
is available from the British Library

ISBN 0 7225 3458 2

Printed in Great Britain by
Caledonian International Book Manufacturing Ltd, Glasgow

Contents

Part III The Recipes

Acknowledgements

I should particularly like to thank aromatherapists Patricia Davis and Frances Clifford for expert help in preparing this book. Thanks are also due to nutritionist Celia Wright, who first opened my eyes to the problem of cellulite, and to masseuse Clare Maxwell-Hudson, for valuable information on the many benefits of massage.

PART I
BANISHING CELLULITE FOREVER

Introduction

It was in 1988 that I first decided to investigate cellulite and cellulite treatments, using myself as a guinea pig. At that time, most people scorned the notion of a special kind of fat which descends on the thighs and bottoms of large numbers of women while mysteriously avoiding male bodies.

Having been plagued by ugly bumps and bulges on my thighs for most of my adult life, I was not convinced by the prevailing orthodoxy which said there was no such thing as cellulite. If it didn't exist, how come I had it?

Since that time the anti-cellulite industry, then in its infancy, has become huge. Most leading cosmetic companies produce anti-cellulite treatments, and newspapers and magazines regularly cover the subject in a serious fashion.

But the public remains almost as confused as ever as to the true nature of cellulite, and many have a sneaking suspicion that it is all so much hype on the part of exploitative beauty companies. At the same time, as bodies become more exposed, ever more women are seeking smooth, slim, sleek thighs, peach-like bottoms and flat stomachs, not just in youth, but throughout their lives.

This is the story of how I managed to lose my own deeply-embedded cellulite, and regain a smooth, trim lower body – by coming to understand the nature of the stuff, and accepting it as an all-too-grim reality.

Like many thousands of other women, I spent most of my adult years hating my lumpy, bumpy, blancmange thighs.

It is not too much of an exaggeration to say that these nasty bulges blighted my life. While they were never life-threatening or a serious health risk, their all-too-obvious presence meant that I was never really able to wear tight jeans, shorts, short skirts, tracksuits or leggings. At least, I always felt I looked a complete fright in anything figure-hugging or leg-revealing. I never felt comfortable in either bikinis or swimming costumes, and never allowed anybody to take pictures of me on the beach. During the days of skintight, flared trousers, the ones supposedly in my size simply wouldn't accommodate my thighs. It may sound amusing now, but it was very upsetting at the time.

The problem was one that only I worried about or took seriously. Other people who knew about my hidden horrors just laughed, and could not understand my preoccupation and worry about something so apparently trivial. My close friends would go out of their way to assure me that I looked perfectly normal, very nice in fact.

But I was not reassured. The 'perfectly normal' appearance was only possible because I went to great lengths (literally) to hide the bumps and bulges. I always wore long skirts, baggy trousers and high-heeled shoes, and took a lot of care over hair and make-up so that attention would be diverted from the guilty secret – the overstuffed sausages I possessed instead of slender thighs.

For a long time, I concluded that my horrible thighs must be just an unfortunate genetic inheritance I could do little about, such as a huge nose or receding chin might be. And yet I knew I hadn't always had such legs. Pictures of me as a child show me with perfectly slim, straight thighs. The acres of dimpled lard descended in late adolescence when I was about fifteen or sixteen and then simply stayed there, weighing me down and making me extremely self-conscious.

But at the back of my mind I never really accepted that nature had intended me to have these lumps and bulges. If so, then she was monstrously unfair, as I couldn't help noticing that not every young woman had them. Although the bulges and dimples were common enough, I could see for myself that they were not an inevitable accompaniment to womanhood. What's more, I wasn't generally fat or overweight. My weight-for-height has always been exactly right according to the tables that are frequently published. All my adult life my thighs have looked as though they belonged to somebody else. I had to put up with fat thighs on an otherwise thin body.

But it wasn't really the girth of my thighs that upset me so much. If they had been merely fat, or well-built, I could have tolerated them more. It was the pockets of fat, the bulges, the jodhpurs, or 'love handles' as they are known in America, that I hated to much. The general appearance was as if somebody had forgotten to say when.

Over the years I tried everything I could to get rid of the bulges and regain the slim, shapely thighs of my pre-adolescence. In fact, most of us with this problem do 'try everything' to slim them down a bit and make them a little more presentable. I went on stringent diets. I did huge amounts of exercise. I went to health farms and submitted myself to saunas, starvation regimes, and endless pummelling and pounding. I went on marathon walks, gave up butter and dairy produce, became vegetarian. I stopped drinking and smoking. I took up yoga, and attempted to contort myself into unlikely positions. As I did so, I could feel the bulges stopping me from attaining the correct postures. It felt like having several bean bags in the way. The only problem was, the bean bags were inside my skin.

While all this effort ensured that I became extremely thin everywhere else, the thigh bulges stayed firmly in place, apparently unbudgeable. Of course, I was a sucker for every 'slim your thighs' book on the market. My friends, knowing about my – to them – needless sensitivity, would buy me thigh-reducing books for Christmas. I also tried the many patent creams which were advertised as having the ability to disperse fat from 'problem areas' such as hips and thighs. Thigh-reducing treatments are still a huge industry – along with all other slimming products.

Needless to say, these creams and lotions didn't even begin to work. Nor did any of the special 'thigh-whittling' exercises which the books recommended. More than ever I became convinced that Mother Nature had doled out these hideous thighs to me as some obscure punishment, to remind me not to get too uppity. I couldn't think what I had done to deserve them, though. Finally, in desperation, I considered plastic surgery or liposuction, where excess fat is vacuumed out of thighs and buttocks.

One look at the before-and-after pictures, though, decided me against this operation. For while the patients had undoubtedly lost inches, *all their bulges and dimples were still there*. Even that drastic measure didn't result in straight, unbumpy thighs.

It was a great relief to me to learn that cosmetic surgery wouldn't solve my problem, because I am a terrible coward and cannot stand any kind of physical pain. Apart from that, these operations are always so very expensive, and can be dangerous.

Now though, all that agonizing, all that hatred directed against my unlovely thighs, is in the past. These days I do not have any lumps or bulges at all. My legs above the knee no longer have an overstuffed look but are the slim, straight limbs I have always coveted. Wonder of wonders, I can now wear tight jeans, tracksuits, bikinis and short skirts if I want to. I am no longer self-conscious about appearing on the beach. I have, at last, been able to accept my thighs as part of me rather than an alien graft, which was how I regarded them before.

When I survey my thighs nowadays I can hardly believe they are mine. In fact, it all seems so much like a dream come true that I often wonder if I will wake up one morning and find that the stuffed mattresses have come back. So far, I'm glad to say, they haven't.

I can't begin to estimate what a difference having thin thighs has made. My self-confidence and self-esteem have shot up and my former self-consciousness has disappeared. I'm quite happy now to wear a leotard or leggings, to reveal my thighs instead of wanting to cover them up and hide them. It's not nice to be desperately ashamed of a part of your body, and my relief at having really quite nice thighs, after two decades of misery over completely unaesthetic ones, is overwhelming.

So what have I done to achieve this miracle? It's quite simple. I came to learn that these bumps and bulges which had so clouded my adult years were not an inherited tendency, nor were they 'womanly curves'. And they were not, in the strict sense of the word, fat.

The dimpled bulges were, in fact, deposits of cellulite, toxic wastes which often accumulate in female fatty tissues and which the body is unable to expel by any usual means.

Theories about cellulite have long been relegated to the cranky, bogus end of the health and beauty scene. The British medical profession has, in recent years, done its best to discredit the notion that poisonous waste can somehow deposit itself on female thighs. And I must admit that when you first hear the idea it does sound pretty implausible. Because the thing is, men don't get cellulite – it's a female-only problem.

Most doctors still maintain that there is no such thing as cellulite, no such thing as a special kind of fat which only women have. If some women do have these bulges on their thighs, well, they just have to learn to put up with them, that's all. Thigh bulges are just tough luck, and really nothing whatever to worry about. They're not an *illness*, for goodness' sake, most doctors will tell you.

Many in the medical profession persist in maintaining that cellulite is a pure invention of cosmetic companies and slimming magazines who want to sell their products and periodicals, and which women are daft enough to believe. Why, even the word itself doesn't exist in the English language. It is a French import, rather like *ooh là là* or *zut alors* – and with about as much meaning for the medical profession. Because we in Britain and America largely don't accept the concept of cellulite we have no word for it. Officially, medically speaking, there's no such thing.

I used to think myself that the idea of cellulite was pure nonsense, something dreamed up by get-rich-quick merchants to play on women's deep-seated fears and insecurities. After all, I didn't want to be considered gullible and naïve. I regarded myself as a sophisticated and cynical journalist, not readily able to have the wool pulled over my eyes.

But when I heard about a treatment which was actually guaranteed to get rid of cellulite, I decided to give it a try. The treatment consisted of a combination of a detoxifying diet, brushing yourself with a hard, scratchy brush made of Mexican cactus, and having aromatherapy oils massaged into the bulges. A few weeks of this regime, I was assured, would make all my cellulite deposits go.

I checked out that the treatments could do no harm, and also that the people offering them were genuine, rather than conwomen just after my money. When I was satisfied on both counts, I became my own guinea pig. I must say, though, that it was in a spirit of the profoundest scepticism that I made my first visit to a nearby aromatherapist. How, I wondered, could her treatments work when everything else, including the most austere of diets, had done nothing to shift the lumps and bumps? And how could she be so sure that cellulite existed, when all the doctors assured me time and again that it was a load of rubbish?

Well, all I can say is that the treatments did work – wonderfully. Nobody was more surprised than I when the lumps and bumps which had been there for two decades, seemingly unshiftable, finally began to soften and eventually disappear altogether. So I wasn't meant to have those bulges after all. Mother Nature hadn't played a cruel trick on me. The deposits were simply waste material that for a long time I hadn't been able to get rid of – and now I had succeeded. The tape measure and other people's comments proved beyond all possible doubt that the ghastly bulges had at long last vanished.

Now when I meet people in the street who haven't seen me for a long time they simply don't recognize me. When they realize who I am their first comment is always: 'Haven't you lost a lot of weight?'

Yet I haven't, really. I've only lost the bulges. The odd thing is that I look far thinner, even in long, bunchy skirts. Some people have told me I now walk differently, more like a fairy than an elephant, as previously. I look lighter, I'm told. And all because the thigh bulges have gone. Because they are not there any more I look like a different person altogether.

Once I embarked on the treatments I investigated the phenomenon of cellulite as thoroughly and scientifically as possible. It's not always easy, making a study of something you have been told categorically doesn't exist. But, I reasoned, that didn't stop Columbus, Galileo and all the other pioneers who have challenged the prevailing orthodoxy. You may say that discovering cellulite isn't as important as knowing whether the world is round, or whether the earth moves round the sun or vice versa. But to me it is. While I can be perfectly happy without any knowledge of geography or astronomy, it is difficult to be completely content with hideous thighs you have to view every single day of your life whether you like it or not.

Anyway, my researches have proved to me that, whatever the doctors say, there is such a thing as cellulite, that it is not the same as ordinary fat, and that there are treatments which will banish it for ever. Doctors don't know everything these days, any more than they ever did.

I believe now that cellulite is an indication of a chronic and possibly quite serious health problem. The deposits are no more supposed to be there than a wart, a verruca or an ingrowing toenail are supposed to be there. The presence of cellulite is an indication that not all is well inside your body.

When I made up my mind to try, finally, to get rid of my lumps and bumps, I enlisted the aid of a professional therapist. In my case this was necessary, as I was still extremely wary of accepting that cellulite existed, and I had to be persuaded by treatments that would work. Also, initially, I knew nothing about the subject, and had to gain information gradually. But it is perfectly possible to treat cellulite all by yourself once you understand what the problem is and why it affects only women.

There is no harm that can come to you from the treatments described in this book, and they have a huge advantage over 'miracle cures' in that they actually do work.

The anti-cellulite programme, in common with most worthwhile things in life, takes quite a bit of dedication and motivation. There's no pill you can swallow to make the cellulite just melt away. Some of the therapies and ideas outlined in this book may seem strange at first, especially as they are unlikely to be endorsed or recommended by your average doctor.

This book is for all those women who have been made miserable by dimpled bulges on their thighs, bulges they thought they had to put up with for all of their lives. Cellulite, I have proved for myself, is not an unavoidable curse of Eve – it is treatable and removable.

You'll not only feel and look far better without the cellulite deposits, your general health will improve as well. Since I got rid of mine I have found that my energy levels have increased considerably. Walking around with those unnecessary bulges was actually making me more tired than I need be.

All I can say is – there is no comparison between life with cellulite and life without it.

Chapter 1

The Evidence for Cellulite

Does cellulite really exist?

This has got to be the first question asked, as very many people, including some who have loads of cellulite, will tell you that it does not, and that it is merely a fancy new word for old-fashioned fat.

Cellulite is the popular name given to those peculiarly female bulges which collect on thighs, buttocks and upper arms, and which go into 'orange-peel' puckers when pressed and squeezed. But if you ask the average British or American doctor about cellulite, you will probably be laughed to scorn and told categorically that there is no such thing. Doctors, on the whole, will tell you that fat is fat and that is that. And there is some basis for their insistence that 'cellulite' is just so much nonsense. The word does not appear in any medical dictionary, and the condition is not described in any English language medical textbook. There has not been, so far as I know, a single clinical trial on the subject. There have been no research papers on cellulite at all, no letters to *The Lancet* about it, and no studies published in any respected medical journal. There is a condition called *cellulitis*, which is the inflammation of cellular tissue when a wound turns septic, but this is a serious condition which bears no relation to the cellulite we are talking about.

Cellulite is a French word which has been adopted by alternative practitioners and beauty therapists simply because there is no other word in the English language to describe the kind of lumpy fat deposits which tend to collect on various parts of the female anatomy.

No doctor can, of course, deny the observable fact that very many women have lumps and bumps on their thighs, and that these bulges do present an 'orange-peel' appearance. But are doctors right in believing that the bulges are formed from exactly the same kind of fat as that found everywhere on our bodies? The average doctor in this country will tell you that under the microscope, there is no difference between the so-called 'cellulite' areas and other fat cells.

But one should not assume that because the existence of cellulite is denied in orthodox medical circles in Britain and America this holds for the rest of the world. In France, the story is very different. Over there, cellulite has been accepted as a genuine medical condition for the past forty years. So much do they accept its existence that you can have anti-cellulite treatments on their equivalent of the National Health Service. French doctors believe that cellulite is not, strictly speaking, fat at all, but a kind of water retention. They believe the condition is caused by the action of female hormones on water and body wastes, and that it can, if untreated, lead to serious health problems such as arthritis.

British doctors are aware that cellulite is something the French take seriously – which is probably one more reason why British medicine gives it short shrift. As late as June 1988 Professor Sam Shuster, consultant dermatologist at the Royal Victoria Infirmary, Newcastle, was referring to cellulite as 'a French load of old cobblers'. His explanation of cellulite was that women have less collagen – the protein which gives skin its thickness – in their bodies than men, and because of this the lumps and bumps are more likely to show through. Men do have these bumps and bulges, according to Shuster, but because their skin is thicker we just don't see them. Professor Shuster wasn't denying the existence of the lumps and bumps – just denying that they could be a type of fat unique to women.

Eugenia Chandris, author of *The Venus Syndrome*, investigated cellulite when trying to understand the reason for her own extremely bottom-heavy shape. She too came rapidly to the conclusion that it was no different from ordinary fat. She writes: 'The cellulite question is not supported by any sound medical evidence. In fact, most doctors disdainfully deny the existence of cellulite: they say it is just ordinary fat. What is the truth?'

Chandris, who eventually resorted to extremely painful plastic surgery to correct her own Christina Onassis-type 'thunder thighs', felt along with Professor Shuster that the only reason we see the stuff on women is because their skin is finer and the lumps and bumps show through more.

Chandris, of Greek origin like Christina Onassis, had been plagued by jodhpur thighs ever since she was a young teenager. Her mother, fearing that such a shape would ruin her chances of making a good marriage, sent her all over the world to try out patent cures and medicines. Nothing worked and, in the end, she seemed to have no choice but to go for plastic surgery.

Her book was published in 1986, many years after the word 'cellulite' first crossed the Channel and the condition was being treated by alternative practitioners.

So who is right? Is there such a thing as cellulite, a women-only type of fat, or is it just something dreamed up by commercial companies who want to make lots of money out of we foolish females? Are all French doctors really talking a load of old cobblers when they accept the existence of cellulite?

Ten years ago, I was as sceptical as most of the British doctors, thinking it was extremely unlikely that there could be a special type of fat which only women possessed. After all, fat cells were fat cells. It was well known that women were predisposed to the pear shape, whereas men tended to be 'apples' and collect fat round their middles. Women became pear-shaped and men got beer bellies. That was an observable difference between the sexes, and both kinds of fat were, it seemed, caused by a combination of over-indulgence in food and drink and under-indulgence in physical activity. Also, it was a fact that metabolism slowed down as people aged, and that middle-aged spread and middle-aged thighs were part of growing older. It was just that differences in anatomy meant that men's and women's fat tended to collect in different places.

Several explanations were offered by the medical profession as to why this happened. One was that female lower body fat served a biological purpose. It was there in case of famine, so that women – who had to reproduce the next generation – would have fat stores for themselves and their unborn babies to feed on, if necessary.

Another explanation was that this type of fat was just an extension of 'womanly curves', which had been provided by nature to make women's bodies soft and appealing, as different as possible from the hard, hairy bodies of men.

A third explanation was that it was the result of gravity. As we got older, obesity experts solemnly assured us, it was only natural that fat would tend to collect in the lower body regions. But this theory, while sounding perfectly logical initially, proved after a minute's thought to be so much nonsense. It could not explain why it was only female thighs that were subject to the laws of gravity. Surely these laws could not be so sexist?

In America, cellulite was seen as a natural, if regrettable, aspect of being a woman. In this country too, we were told by people such as romantic novelist Barbara Cartland that we should not attempt to get rid of this fat, as men liked something 'to grab hold of'.

Although I and very many other women had little choice but to accept these theories, there remained at the back of my mind a nagging doubt. Having been assured time and time again that cellulite did not exist I could not quite understand why I should see it so clearly every time I glanced down at my naked thighs. I had been told that this was just ordinary fat, but if so, why did it collect only in certain places? And why was it that no dieting or exercise regimes did anything to diminish the dimples?

It didn't take tremendous powers of observation for me to see for myself that many women who had cellulite were not otherwise fat. There was, quite clearly, something that was different about it. There had to be some good reason, too, why only women collected bulgy fat on their thighs, and men never did.

However much we were told that cellulite did not exist we still didn't like it being there. So when patent anti-cellulite treatments began appearing on the market in the mid-seventies (most of them hailing from France) we fell for them.

Of course, British doctors lost no time in warning us against these patent cures, saying that there was no evidence whatever that they could work to melt fat away from thighs. The very existence of these creams, concocted, the manufacturers told us, from precious herbal extracts distilled by a mysterious process, seemed to give credence to the medical profession's firmly held conviction that the concept of cellulite had been invented by cosmetic companies to foist yet another unnecessary product onto the ever-gullible consumer. All you had to do, the doctors cynically observed, was to play on female vanity and you had a licence to print money.

These new anti-cellulite creams were beguilingly advertised and presented. The message was that they were specially designed to rid problem areas of ugly lumps and bumps. The products were always illustrated with a picture of a beautiful young woman blessed with the slenderest thighs, the implication being that a diligent application of the cream could give you the same kind of enviable legs.

I wanted to believe the claims made by the manufacturers of these creams, but common sense seemed to tell me that they couldn't possibly work. It appeared most likely that they belonged in exactly the same category as hair restorers, bust enlargers and pills to restore sexual potency and attractiveness. In other words, they were preying on universal fears ripe for exploitation by the get-rich-quick merchants since the beginning of time.

Of course, the products didn't even begin to work. Those of us who tried them found that however hard we rubbed them in, the lumps and bumps remained as firmly in place as ever. So of course more than ever we seemed to have no choice but to believe the doctors who assured us that cellulite was an invention by those dastardly Frogs, who believed they could foist anything on a naive and unsuspecting British public.

Before long, the Advertising Standards Authority stepped in to say that the claims made for most of these creams and lotions were unsupported by any scientific evidence and should be withdrawn. As a result, the claims that these products could magically melt away fat, themselves melted away and were replaced by more innocuous wording, such as that they could 'improve circulation'. Well, you couldn't argue about the ability of a cream to improve circulation if you rubbed it in vigorously enough.

Most of these products stayed on the market, however, although sales must have been adversely affected. But the fact that these highly expensive French creams sold at all highlights the despair of millions of women who know they have lumpy, bulging thighs that they hate, whatever the doctors say.

Then, around 1981, came a breakthrough in my own understanding of the problem, enabling me to view cellulite in a completely new way. I was asked by a newspaper to write an article on the subject, pulling together all the latest views and theories. The controversy over whether it did or did not exist had reared up again, for some reason. As expected, all the doctors and obesity experts I consulted reiterated their belief that cellulite was a figment of hysterical women's imagination.

This time I didn't leave it there. I contacted Celia Wright, who with her husband Brian was running a forward-thinking nutrition centre in Sussex. Celia and Brian had both spent many years investigating and trying out all the new theories on nutrition and health, and approached everything completely open-mindedly. To them, any theory is innocent until proved guilty.

Celia firmly believed that cellulite did exist and that it was not merely something dreamed up by French cosmetic companies with French franc signs in their eyes. 'As I see it,' she told me, 'cellulite isn't really fat at all in the strict sense of the word. It's actually toxic waste material that the body cannot get rid of in the ordinary way, and has dumped to far-off sites, well out of the way of vital organs.'

She further explained that the reason only women suffer from cellulite is a hormonal one, recognized by French doctors all those years ago. The female hormone oestrogen, said Celia, acts to send toxins to thighs, buttocks and upper arms because it has a protective as well as a reproductive function. Oestrogen works to protect vital organs in case of pregnancy. Men don't get cellulite because there is not the same vital need to protect their bodies from collecting rubbish. Whereas women get cellulite, men get furred-up arteries. (It is actually medically known that oestrogen protects women from coronary heart disease, and that this is why women usually succumb to heart attacks only after the menopause, when oestrogen is no longer circulating.)

I had never heard this explanation before but instantly it began to make sense. If cellulite is, as Celia said, accumulated toxic waste rather than real fat, it would explain why no amount of dieting and exercise would ever shift the stuff. If oestrogen plays an important part in the formation of cellulite, this could be the reason why only women get it.

It would also shed light on male doctors' persistent denial of the existence of cellulite. Of course they often are not particularly interested in female-only problems.

So why is it, I asked Celia Wright, that the body cannot eliminate these so-called toxins? (You have to remember that even in the early 1980s most doctors laughed at the idea that the human body could harbour 'toxins' for years on end. Their view was that the body was perfectly well-equipped with organs of elimination, and that no modern diets were poisonous, anyway.)

Celia explained that in normal circumstances the body's own waste disposal system does an excellent job. The problem is that these days many of us overload our bodies with processed foods, coffee, alcohol, cigarettes, environmental pollution – and in the end, the system simply can't cope. It does its best, but there is sometimes just too much waste for it to handle. The main reason why cellulite stays in place, she added, and is so very difficult to get rid of, is that once the body sends the rubbish to thighs, buttocks and upper arms it reckons it has done its job of waste disposal. So it forgets all about the stuff and makes no further effort to shift it.

After I had heard Celia's theory, I began to read books and articles on the subject by other nutritional experts, such as Leslie Kenton and herbalist Kitty Campion. They were all saying exactly the same things about cellulite – that it wasn't real fat, that it was a waste disposal problem, and that it was caused by eating the wrong kinds of food and living the wrong kind of lifestyle, rather than by simply eating too much and taking too little exercise.

It seemed to me that either these women were just repeating each other's cranky theories, or they knew something that doctors didn't. The difficulty, of course, was that none of them is a qualified doctor – Celia Wright and Leslie Kenton are entirely self-taught, and Kitty Campion has trained as a herbalist, which is a speciality not widely recognized by conventional doctors.

Alternative practitioners had always maintained that cellulite did exist. But until the alternative medicine revolution of the eighties, these practitioners were held in low esteem by the medical profession. Now, with the interest in the relationship between diet and health and natural therapies, they began to come into their own, and people began to take what they had to say more seriously.

After studying the subject properly and listening to what alternative therapists had to say on the subject I came to the definite conclusion that cellulite exists. The toxic waste explanation made far more sense than any other I had heard, and in addition it accorded perfectly with all the new ideas on health and nutrition which were being increasingly accepted by open-minded people.

By turning myself into my own guinea pig I have proved conclusively to my own satisfaction that cellulite is a different problem from ordinary fat. Whereas once I was plagued with acres of the stuff, now I have none at all. I did not find any scientific or medical papers on the subject, and it was only when I accepted the 'alternative' explanation and tried the 'alternative' treatments that my cellulite began to disappear.

However, even now most British doctors are denying the existence of cellulite. By and large, they have not been persuaded. This is what Dr David Delvin, a well-known media doctor and 'agony uncle' to several women's magazines, has to say about it, writing in the doctors' journal *General Practitioner* in May 1988: 'Many people have great difficulty in losing an excessive bulge from their bottoms. As you probably know, women's magazines and beauty clinics tend to promote the idea that these bulges are extremely hard to shift because they contain a mysterious substance called cellulite.

'Personally, I don't know of any evidence that cellulite actually *exists* – and you certainly won't find it in the pages of Muir's *Pathology* textbook.'

I'm inclined to think that Muir (presumably a man) might learn something if he listened to herbalists, aromatherapists and holistic healers. They are convinced that cellulite does exist, and that it is an eminently treatable condition – without resorting to painful and expensive cosmetic surgery.

In his article, Dr Delvin went on to say that the 'orange-peel' fat can be removed by a horrific-sounding surgical operation which is extremely painful and 'fairly drastic'.

But it's not at all necessary. Once you accept that cellulite is a visible sign that the body is harbouring toxic wastes, you can then embark on treatments which enable the poisons to disperse, rather than using the surgeon's knife to slice it away.

Chapter 2

The Causes of Cellulite

I think we can safely assume that cellulite does exist, whatever some doctors may say to the contrary, and that it is a major problem for thousands of women in the world today.

Every woman who has cellulite would rather not have it. But having been assured by countless medical 'experts' that the stuff doesn't exist, the cellulite sufferer has assumed it is just something she has to put up with, just another of the difficulties which go with being a woman.

This is not so. Nature never meant us to have cellulite and we would all be a lot better off without it. But before attempting any successful anti-cellulite regime it is essential to understand exactly what cellulite is, why it develops, and what will make it go away. It becomes possible to get rid of it once you understand why it forms.

So how do you know whether you've got cellulite in the first place? One of the main characteristics is dimples. You know you've got cellulite on your legs if they have a dimply appearance when you stand up. Another factor is that cellulite areas feel cold to the touch. This is because circulation is poor in those areas.

Almost always, the skin on cellulite areas is whiter and more difficult to tan than other skin.

Cellulite is not flab, and it is not fat. Flabby skin does not have the dimpled appearance, and nor does ordinary fat. If you pinch an area containing cellulite you will find that it stays up for far longer than skin pinched, say, on the forearm. This indicates that the fat cells are waterlogged. If it is allowed to accumulate, it becomes hard and grainy. In the early stages it is soft because of the presence of fluid, but becomes progressively harder as the years go by. The harder cellulite is, the more difficult it becomes to lose, although it is never impossible.

The presence of cellulite is nothing to do with being overweight. You can be verging on anorexia and still have cellulite deposits. Conversely, you can be extremely fat and still not have any cellulite on your legs.

If you do have it, though, you should do all you can to get rid of the stuff. For it indicates that your body is in a toxic condition. If the cellulite is left untreated, the toxicity could lead to more serious conditions, such as arthritis or permanent water retention. The presence of cellulite is a warning that your body needs a thorough cleanse and detoxification.

THE DISCOVERY OF CELLULITE

Is cellulite a new problem, brought about by the artificiality of modern living, or has it always existed? Of course, it is difficult to be certain, as the concept and treatment did not come into being until about forty years ago. But, looking at certain Old Master paintings, it seems as though cellulite certainly existed in the seventeenth century. Many of the nudes in Rubens' paintings, for instance, seem to have loads of cellulite. Patricia Davis, who was one of the first British aromatherapists to develop a successful cellulite treatment, believes that it is not a new phenomenon at all.

'Most of Rembrandt's nude paintings were of his second wife – and boy, did she have cellulite,' Patricia said. 'All the characteristics are there – the dimpliness, the whiteness, the bulges. The classic painting of a woman with cellulite is the one where she is stepping into water semi-nude, and you just see the texture of her thighs, which are a dead giveaway.

'It seems extremely reasonable to suppose that cellulite existed in Holland in the sixteenth and seventeenth centuries. After all, the Dutch diet was high in dairy produce and the rich women would have led extremely sedentary lives. So I doubt that it's all that new, although few people would have bothered about it much when thighs were never normally exposed.'

Patricia Davis says that she first became aware of cellulite as a medical problem in France around 1952, when she was studying ballet there. 'At that time, the condition was attributed to water retention, and was considered treatable,' she said. 'In fact, we now know that although cellulite and water retention are linked, they are not exactly the same thing.

'The standard treatment in those days was hydrotherapy at one of the famous spas, where extremely fierce jets of water would be applied to the affected areas. Hydrotherapy is the medicinal equivalent to a jacuzzi. The treatment worked, because you got a lot of pummelling, which would drive the cellulite out of the fat cells and help it to disperse. This treatment was backed up by lots of ordinary massage, mud baths and a "nature cure" diet.

'In the 1950s the condition was thought to be caused by poor kidney function, which meant that excess water could not be excreted. Now of course, we know that cellulite is caused by a sluggish lymphatic system. But certainly in France it was always recognized as a woman-only problem.'

Patricia became interested in the question of diet and health when, at the early age of twenty-six, she developed severe arthritis. She gave up dancing when her first child was born, and soon her arthritis was so bad that she could not even walk down the street.

'My doctor told me that I had given up dancing too quickly, and that arthritis was always a danger for dancers and athletes who suddenly stop. I was put on some drugs which were later found to be highly dangerous, but the condition just got worse. In those days – 1956 – nobody ever spoke about curing yourself through diet. It would have been considered extremely cranky.

'But one day a friend said, "Why don't you try the nature cure?" She lent me a book written in the 1930s, and everything I read made complete sense. I put myself straightaway on what we would now call a healthy diet, and cured my own arthritis completely. Since going on the nature cure I have never had even a twinge.

'That opened my eyes to the powerful effect food can have on bodies. Having made myself completely symptom-free I helped other people with arthritis, and then realized I could treat those with chronic illnesses.'

When her children were young Patricia ran a ballet school, but later she trained as an aromatherapist and masseuse and set up business in the mid 1960s. It was then that she began to realize the extent of the cellulite problem. In those days, she said, women did not come to her for their cellulite, as most had no idea they were suffering from any kind of treatable condition. They just assumed that the lumps and bumps were some-how supposed to be there, just the way they were made.

'Very many of my clients were coming to me because of a weight problem, ' she said. 'But as I mas-saged them, I realized that many hadn't got a weight problem at all but were suffering from cellulite instead.

I would tell them that it wasn't fat they had, but cellulite, and they would say: but what's that?'

Since there were no textbooks to guide her, Patricia Davis began treating cellulite with hard massage and essential oils. 'It was simply trial and error,' she told me. 'I knew from my aromatherapy training that certain essential oils did help the body to cleanse and detoxify, and that others were stimulating for circulation. The effect of certain essential oils has been very well documented in France, and I simply applied this knowledge to the cellulite problem.

'I knew all about detoxifying diets from treating my own arthritis, and so I just put the two bits of knowledge together. If, as I suspected, cellulite was a toxic condition, then the diet plus massage and aromatherapy treatments would get rid of it. And of course, it did.

'But I have to say that I and other aromatherapists were proceeding very much from theory. In the early days, it was a matter of backing a hunch, as we had no medical textbooks to guide us. It was all very difficult, as our treatments and suggestions were being completely derided by orthodox doctors, who regarded us as charlatans and cranks.'

In many ways, the story of cellulite can be compared to the pre-menstrual tension saga. In the 1920s and 1930s there was no mention whatever of PMT in any medical textbook. So far as the mainly male medical profession was concerned, the condition simply didn't exist. All 'female problems' were just evidence that women were the weaker sex and had to be humoured and pacified like children. And of course, all doctors knew the correct cure for period problems of any kind – go away and have a baby.

It wasn't until gynaecologist Dr Katharina Dalton began to ask pertinent questions about hormonal fluctuations in women that the syndrome began to be recognized, named, and written up in medical literature. This was in 1953. When Dr Dalton began training as a doctor she was already married with three children, and had noticed that whenever she became pregnant the headaches, depression, heaviness and bloating that she suffered from just before a period, went away. Of course, in those days, the term 'premenstrual tension' had not been invented. But through study and research, Dr Dalton came to realize that it was a medical condition suffered by very many women, and that it was treatable.

Now, of course, her conclusions are accepted by all doctors, several of which have set up special PMT clinics. PMT is big business nowadays, and huge sums of money are being made out of patent treatments such as evening primrose oil and vitamin B_6. Consequently it is hard to realize that only forty years ago doctors were assuring women there was no such thing as PMT. Problems associated with menstruation were, like many women-only complaints, seen as trivial.

Over the past few years there has been much research on PMT. Since about 1980 it has been established that there is a definite connection between PMT and the lack of certain vitamins, minerals and essential fatty acids. This explosion of knowledge on the subject means that there is no longer any reason for women to suffer from PMT – at least, not in silence.

The same thing now needs to happen with cellulite. Unlike PMT, which comes and goes, cellulite is an ever-present problem. There is plenty of evidence to suggest that it is caused by the wrong kind of diet, stress, prescription drugs, a sedentary lifestyle, too much tea, coffee and alcohol, cigarettes, poor circulation and a sluggish lymphatic system.

Although cellulite has probably always existed, it seems reasonable to suppose that the problem is getting worse. The main reason for this is that more women than ever now smoke, drink, eat processed foods and take prescription drugs, such as the pill. All of these alter hormonal balance and may well affect the workings of vital organs.

The other factor which has a bearing on our new awareness of cellulite is that it is only in the latter half of this century that women generally began exposing their legs and thighs. In the past, that was confined to artists' models. In the mid-1960s, with the advent of miniskirts, the standard explanation of bulgy thighs was that they were caused by cold weather. If girls were daft enough to walk around in the middle of winter with skirts halfway up their thighs they must expect some bulges, doctors seriously said.

They then explained cellulite by saying that the body developed extra layers of fat to cope with the cold. For a time, we all believed this. But then when miniskirts went out of fashion to be replaced by midi skirts and the bulges still didn't go away, that theory fell into disuse.

To me, the most telling evidence for the existence of cellulite is the neat appearance of French women over 'a certain age'. Whereas the majority of middle-aged English women have thighs absolutely thick with cellulite, it is noticeably absent from the legs of French ladies. Now, either French women are constructed completely differently from their English counterparts, or they have learned something that we still need to learn – that cellulite is a problem which can be treated.

Not that cellulite is a problem confined to older women by any means. The condition can appear as early as the age of twelve or thirteen and then remain for life, unless treated.

HOW DO WE GET CELLULITE, AND WHY?

Cellulite is a problem confined to women. Men never get it. As such, it is safe to assume that there is a hormonal factor involved. In fact, it seems most likely – and I have to say 'seems' because there are no proper medical studies on the subject – that the condition is caused, above all, by the presence of oestrogen.

The more oestrogen there is in a woman's body, the more likely it is that cellulite will develop. The danger times for developing cellulite are at puberty, pregnancy and the menopause, the times of greatest hormonal fluctuation.

Cellulite was first thought to have a hormonal component when French doctors realized that men never suffered from it. It was then discovered that the female hormone oestrogen predisposes women towards retaining fluid. From there, it was a short step towards an understanding that oestrogen must somehow be implicated in the formation of cellulite.

Unless women are frequently pregnant, they have high levels of oestrogen circulating around their system continuously. The amount of oestrogen circulating in women's bodies has also increased enormously since the mid 1960s with the introduction of the contraceptive pill and hormone replacement therapy for post-menopausal women.

Oestrogen has a specific purpose, and that is to prepare the body to receive and nurture an embryo. Whenever pregnancy occurs, the amount of oestrogen circulating in the system drops rapidly. Nowadays most women have far more oestrogen circulating in their system than was intended by nature. It acts to send waste materials away from vital organs and into areas where they will be relatively harmless. This eventually becomes apparent as cellulite. In men, waste products have the effect of furring up their arteries, so they are more likely to succumb to heart attacks. It seems as if biology acts to protect the female. We get cellulite, whereas men get hardening of the arteries – a condition which is taken extremely seriously by most doctors. What they have not realized yet is that cellulite and coronary heart disease are different manifestations of an identical problem – too much stress, a bad diet, too little exercise, and too much rubbish getting into the system and not being able to get out.

Although men don't have cellulite some of them do have beer bellies, which are a related problem caused mainly by the high oestrogen content of hops. It is also noticeable that men who are very heavy beer drinkers often suffer from female-type breast development. This is yet another indication that oestrogen appears to predispose towards the retention of unwanted fluid.

Recent studies on the contraceptive pill have linked it with the formation of breast cancer and an increased incidence of thrombosis. Dr Ellen Grant, an early researcher into oral contraception and now one of the pill's most outspoken opponents, believes that it is linked with general bad health in women. She argues that the pill significantly interferes with carbohydrate metabolism and blood function. Studies carried out by Professor Victor Wynn at the metabolic unit, St Mary's Hospital, in London, have shown that the pill encourages blood fats to increase. It also stops the uptake of certain essential minerals such as zinc, iron and magnesium, and encourages an excess of copper to stay in the system.

Dr Grant does not mention in her book *The Bitter Pill* that oral contraception encourages the formation of cellulite, but from what we know about the action of oestrogen it seems extremely likely that this is so. Although cellulite is very probably not a new problem, as far as we can tell it appears to be far more prevalent in the late twentieth century than at any other time in history.

The contraceptive pill is, of course, formulated from synthetic hormones. But the body does not distinguish between synthetic and natural hormones, and so far as the female system is concerned, taking the pill simply means that the oestrogen action on the body is increased.

Ellen Grant believes that oral contraceptives interfere with body metabolism and the release of complex biochemical substances. They can also cause far-reaching blood and circulatory changes and can lead to weight gain and breast tenderness.

Another factor, most probably linked to hormones, is that women's bodies simply cannot take the same amount of punishment and abuse that men's can. We know now for a fact that women's tolerance threshold for alcohol and nicotine is far lower than men's. But all the time women are abusing their bodies, oestrogen performs its powerful protective function, and does its best to send the waste to outlying areas so that we will survive.

The reason most of us don't feel ill when we have a cellulite problem is that the body has been successful in sending the rubbish far away from vital organs. With men, the rubbish is retained nearer the centre, which is why they are far more likely to suffer from heart, circulatory and blood pressure problems.

To sum up, we can say that cellulite forms when there is a general circulatory problem in the body. It is, above all, an indication of a sluggish circulation, a sign that body wastes cannot be disposed of in the normal way. When cellulite is present, this means that the lymphatic system, the body's main vacuum cleaner, cannot do its job, and that there is internal clogging.

The next step is to understand exactly what causes the clogging in the first place. Because once this is understood, we can set about unclogging the system.

THE MAIN CAUSES OF CELLULITE

There is very little we can do to decrease the amount of oestrogen circulating in our bodies. But oestrogen will not send rubbish to outlying areas unless there is rubbish to send. So the first thing to understand about cellulite is that it is caused mainly by leading the wrong lifestyle. The body is very clever at recognizing the difference between nutrients and anti-nutrients, and does all it can to neutralize the effect of those substances which it does not need, and which actually have a harmful effect.

COFFEE

Of all cellulite-causing substances, probably the most harmful is coffee, because of the caffeine it contains. The bad effects of coffee have now been well documented, and several medical studies have suggested that more than three cups a day can do damage. None of the studies mentions cellulite, of course, as a possible adverse side-effect of caffeine, but the substance has now been definitely linked with all kinds of female complaints from benign breast lumps to pelvic disorders. Caffeine interferes with the uptake of certain essential minerals in the diet, particularly iron, and also predisposes to certain anxiety states.

The main reason for this is that caffeine puts extra stress on the adrenal glands, which release adrenaline. Like cocaine, caffeine gives the system an instant boost by making the adrenals pump out extra adrenaline. The problem is that when we drink huge amounts of coffee, we enable large quantities of adrenaline to be released which are not burned up at all. Biologically, adrenaline exists to protect us from danger, to enable us to run away or to stay and fight. We naturally get surges of adrenaline when there is a near miss on the motorway, when we are about to take an important exam or attend a vital interview. Then, when the danger is past, the adrenaline production ceases. Caffeine enables this hormone to be secreted all the time.

So coffee puts extra stress on the adrenals by over-working them. They discharge too much adrenaline into the system and become exhausted. Too much caffeine in the system also puts extra stress onto the kidneys, where all water-soluble rubbish is taken so that the blood can be cleansed.

It is now well known that a high intake of caffeine puts people at extra risk of heart attack, as it increases the amount of cholesterol in the system. This causes even more clogging up. In women, the net result of over-consumption is to increase the amount of cellulite on the thighs. For most women, the presence of cellulite is a potent indicator that they are drinking too much caffeine, in the form of tea, coffee, or colas. Chocolate also contains a significant amount of caffeine.

Drinks containing caffeine make you feel good by giving you an instant lift, but this is followed not much later by a nasty low – the well-known withdrawal symptoms. In women who are pregnant or on the pill, caffeine is eliminated particularly slowly, which indicates a hormonal link.

Furthermore, coffee beans are loaded with pesticides, which in large quantities can upset the digestive process. There is no particular advantage in drinking tea, either, as it also contains significant amounts of caffeine, though only half as much as coffee and, in addition, can be loaded with impurities such as copper. Consuming anti-nutrients means that the deposits of cellulite can only get bigger.

In the past, both women and men would have drunk very little coffee. It was first introduced into the Western world in the eighteenth century, and for a long time was confined to men drinking it occasionally in the famous coffee houses. It was not until the 1920s that women began to drink coffee every day, and the development of instant coffee – even worse for you than the filtered variety – meant that we could all drink vast amounts every day.

Now, of course, coffee is the favourite non-alcoholic beverage among young women. Very many women also drink vast quantities of tea, thinking nothing of downing five or six cups a day.

Possibly one of the reasons the French recognized cellulite so long ago was that they have for a long time been a nation of dedicated coffee-drinkers. Coffee and tea have now become our most universal stimulants, and we tend to forget that, delicious though they may be, they are actually non-nutrients, substances the body emphatically does not need for its daily functioning.

The potentially addictive quality of tea and coffee is a warning sign, or should be. The body develops specific cravings only when its biochemistry has been artificially adapted to accommodate an alien substance. If you give your body just what it needs for proper functioning, cravings and addictions do not develop. Unfortunately, in our present society, we have mistaken cravings and addictions for excitement. We appear to thrive on artificial sensual stimulation, forgetting that the human body was not originally designed to cope with these substances. It is hardly surprising if, after a time, it cannot cope with the onslaught and starts to rebel.

Of course, not everybody who consumes vast quantities of caffeine will get cellulite any more than every single person who smokes will die of lung cancer. Some systems can withstand large amounts of stimulating beverages, others can't. The fact is, though, that caffeine significantly adds to the burden on the body.

NICOTINE

Nicotine, like caffeine, is extremely bad for women. It is bad for men as well, but it seems that a woman's system is less able to withstand the poisons released by tobacco in the blood-stream. We have known for twenty years or more that smoking during pregnancy causes low-birthweight babies and, more recently, it has also been linked with malformations and brain damage in embryos.

The first effect of nicotine is that it uses up oxygen, reducing the amount available for use by the cells. It does this by decreasing the efficiency of the lungs. It also affects the haemoglobin – red cells – in the blood. Haemoglobin is the main carrier for oxygen in the blood, and picks up the oxygen in the lungs as the blood circulates.

If the oxygen exchange in the blood is less efficient because of nicotine intake, then every cell in the body will receive less oxygen than it should. This factor is extremely relevant to the cellulite problem because, above all, oxygen acts as a powerful stimulator and cleanser for the blood. Body cells cannot function without adequate oxygen any more than we can ourselves. Whenever there is reduced oxygen in the body, cell function is impaired and circulation is adversely affected.

Some anti-cellulite therapists in America are now noticing that the problem is worse in young girls than in middle-aged women. The main reason for this, they theorize, is increased cigarette consumption. Because although older women – and men – are now significantly reducing their nicotine intake, the habit is becoming more prevalent among young people.

A recent large-scale study among schoolchildren in Britain revealed that teenage girls are now smoking far more than teenage boys. In addition, they find it more difficult to give up, and are more likely to become addicted smokers by the time they are in their mid-twenties. The main reasons given for taking up the habit were release of tension, and a desire to appear sophisticated, 'cool' and grown up.

Smoking adds to the amount of toxic wastes that enter the body, which means that the system has to work even harder to get rid of them. Nicotine is a powerful pollutant and, like caffeine, it is an anti-nutrient.

Its effect is to rob the system of essential substances such as Vitamin C and zinc.

A report by the Royal College of Physicians in 1983 provides some useful figures on women and smoking. Few women, according to the report, smoked before the Second World War but by 1956 around forty-two per cent of women in Britain aged sixteen and over were smokers. Since that time, there has been a steady decline, with around thirty-seven per cent of British women smoking today. The vast majority of these are women under the age of twenty-five.

It has been known for decades that women who smoke are at vastly increased risk from heart disease and all diseases of the circulatory system. It has also now been established that smoking affects fertility and results in an earlier menopause.

The Royal College's report states that women seem to find it harder than men to give up smoking, and adds that the reason for this is unclear. One major reason why women continue to smoke is that they are afraid of gaining weight if they give up. Smoking increases metabolism, and also provides an alternative to eating when some kind of comfort is needed. But as smoking affects circulation, it also adds to cellulite deposits which are, of course, as much a problem as overweight.

The anti-cellulite programme outlined in this book ensures that smoking can be given up without any danger at all of unwelcome weight gain.

ALCOHOL

As with cigarettes and coffee, alcohol consumption was not a significant factor for women until the 1920s, the so-called 'flapper age' when cocktails became popular and it was suddenly fashionable for women to drink. Nowadays, most women drink alcohol regularly.

Women can take far less alcohol than men. One reason for this is that female livers are smaller and able to process less. Another reason is that women's bodies have a higher proportion of fat than men's, and alcohol does not enter fat cells. This means that its effect is concentrated into a smaller area and takes longer to be processed by the liver.

Alcohol enters the blood very quickly and instantly alters blood chemistry. It adds to the workload of the liver, which can then very quickly become overloaded. When alcohol is added to the sum total of non-nutrients entering the body the result is that the liver and kidneys cannot effectively handle the excess waste material. For most people, the eliminative organs have enough to do handling ordinary waste materials produced by the diet. If they have to deal with caffeine, nicotine and alcohol loads as well it is not surprising that they find it hard to cope, and that much waste matter simply stays in the system.

DIET

Although deposits of cellulite can be seen clearly in the paintings of Rubens, Rembrandt and Renoir, it is unlikely that women living in pre-literate societies ever collected much of the stuff. In fact, very few women living what we might call a 'natural' life – eating wholefoods, lots of fruit and vegetables and not drinking tea, coffee or alcohol – ever develop a cellulite problem.

In the modern West, the eliminative difficulties caused by smoking, coffee and alcohol consumption are exacerbated by an artificial diet. In recent years we have of course been urged to eat more fruit and vegetables, brown rice and wholemeal bread in order to stave off serious diseases. Nutritionists say that we were designed to eat a pure, wholefood diet and to experience stress only at certain times, such as when specific dangers threatened. We have already seen how a high caffeine intake adds to the number of stress hormones circulating round the body. Excess stress is also placed on body systems by eating artificial and processed foods, substances which, like caffeine and alcohol, the body was not designed to cope with.

When a pure, natural diet is eaten, the liver and large intestine are extremely efficient at getting rid of wastes very quickly. In fact, the more natural the food, the quicker the digestive system breaks it down. The more artificial it becomes, the longer it takes to go through the body. In some cases, the artificial substance may not be eliminated by the body at all, and may simply stay in the system, sometimes for years on end. Recent work in America on colon cleansing – which is very similar to the anti-cellulite programme – revealed that years of eating artificial foods mean that waste products are never eliminated from the colon but remain there for ever. Autopsies nowadays often reveal many pounds of waste material which would have been completely eliminated if the system had been working effectively.

Much of the waste material that is not handled by the liver or large intestine gets reabsorbed back into the body, where it starts to do damage. It is when too much waste material accumulates that we notice cellulite deposits. The more the system is clogged up and the more sluggish the circulation becomes, the worse the cellulite problem is likely to be.

Cellulite-encouraging foodstuffs are sugar, dairy produce, meat and anything processed, smoked or preserved. Sugar has a similar effect on the body to caffeine, in that it releases adrenalin and gives a quick energy boost, followed by a 'down' not long after. Dairy produce is mucus-forming, which means that it encourages waste material to become sticky and stay in the system. Meat products also take a long time to be processed by the body and, in some cases, may never be entirely eliminated.

WATER

These days, most people do not drink enough water. Very many people never drink any at all, and imagine that diet colas, fruit juices and 'health drinks' do much the same job, or that herbal teas are 'better' for you than black tea.

In fact, water is the only drink which can successfully rehydrate the body, and help to flush out toxins and accumulated wastes from the system. *No other drink can do this*. In fact, whenever you have a drink which is not water, award it minus points, and make sure you have a glass of water to compensate for it. We need to drink at least a litre of water a day, in water form – not in other liquids. Remember, nothing which is not water counts as water. This is most important for all cellulite sufferers.

A SEDENTARY LIFESTYLE

Women who are very active eat a wholefood diet and abstain from alcohol, cigarettes and caffeine, will rarely get cellulite. These days, very many women have jobs that necessitate sitting at a desk all day long. Prolonged inactivity of this kind can cut off circulation. When treating cellulite, therapists often notice that cellulite deposits are at their most intractable where the legs meet the chair edge – at the place where circulation is cut off most.

Prolonged physical inactivity leads to an increasingly sluggish circulation, making it even harder for the blood and lymphatic system to get rid of waste materials and send life-giving oxygen round the system.

HOW CELLULITE FORMS

Cellulite is, above all, a signal that the body's circulation is slowing down and becoming ineffective. Research carried out in Italy shows clearly that cellulite cells are different from other fat cells. Definite physical changes take place in the cells resulting in enlarged capillaries and a weakening of the capillary walls.

The diagrams (a) and (b) show what happens when fat cells are invaded by cellulite. Diagram (a) shows normal, cellulite-free fat cells, with thin capillaries. Diagram (b) shows the effects of cellulite. The capillaries have become greatly enlarged, and blood plasma has seeped out of them into the surrounding fatty tissue. This causes the fat cells to bunch up together, rather than being widely separated as in the first diagram. The effect of this is that the lymph nodes, which normally would drain away excess fluid, become unable to cope, and so the excess plasma stays in the cells.

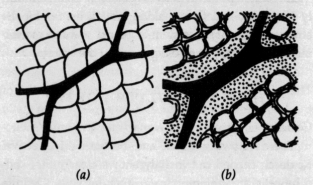

(a)   *(b)*

At the same time as all this is happening, the walls of the fat cells change their structure, to become thickened by extra deposits of collagen. When this takes place, there is further congestion of the circulation, resulting in even more cellulite. So, whenever you have some cellulite, conditions are always created for more to form. The fatty cells become waterlogged and toxin-loaded, full of junk the body simply cannot eliminate.

Cellulite forms when women's bodies produce or take in too much oestrogen, resulting in waste matter being pushed away from vital organs. At the same time as this increased oestrogen pushes the waste away, we are taking in too much junk in the form of food residues, chemicals, artificial additives and preservatives, nicotine, alcohol and tobacco.

As the body was not designed to cope with all these non-nutrients it simply does not know what to do with them. Although the liver can detoxify a certain amount of hormones out of the blood, and keep the bloodstream relatively clear, it cannot manage vastly increased amounts of oestrogen. Nor can it cope with the daily onslaught of junk foods and junk substances. There is no biological mechanism to rid our bodies of the huge amount of junk and pollution which daily invade them.

There are basically two kinds of junk the body has to deal with – the water-soluble kind and the fat-soluble kind. The kidneys handle the former, and the liver looks after the latter. If all the waste material which enters our bodies had to be coped with by the liver we would become seriously ill with liver-related problems. As it is, women are protected by the mechanisms that send the rubbish to out-of-the-way places.

This is the main reason why, although we speak of cellulite 'sufferers', very few of them are ever conscious of the process. They cannot feel the cellulite being formed but are very aware of the unsightly bumps once they have appeared – and they will certainly experience pain when undergoing the kind of hard massage needed to get rid of intractable deposits. But usually cellulite sufferers feel just the same as any other women. This is because our hormonal structure has acted to protect us in a way that it does not protect men. Patricia Davis says: 'The formation of cellulite is really nature protecting those who have to reproduce the species. A lot of poisons get locked in fatty cells, but this is far better for the system than that they should be trapped in the liver, kidneys or arteries.' She defines cellulite as 'a state in which the cells of the subcutaneous fatty layer are invaded by watery deposits carrying toxic waste matter ... Poor circulation of the blood and a sluggish lymphatic system underlie this condition, and women who have a sedentary job or lifestyle and take little or no exercise are those most often affected.'

The other factor, says Davis, is a diet high in toxic substances – tea, coffee and alcohol, red meats, animal fats and foods containing additives such as artificial colours, flavourings, preservatives or emulsifying chemicals. Smoking is another toxic risk, and living or working in an atmosphere laden with other people's smoke can be almost as bad.

'When a high level of toxins in the body is found jointly with a poor circulation,' she adds, 'the conditions exist in which cellulite can develop. Circulation becomes sluggish in the affected areas, so not enough life-giving oxygen can reach the cells from the blood. At the same time, toxins lodge in the cells because the flow of blood is not sufficient to carry them away. The lymphatic system becomes overworked and cannot drain the cell fluid away effectively. And so, gradually, the whole area becomes stagnant.'

I don't need any further proof to tell me that cellulite exists. Do you?

I believe that the main reason doctors continue to deny the existence of cellulite is that they have no treatments at all to deal with it. There are no pills which will send it away, and diuretics, which are often prescribed to people with a water retention problem, can result in serious losses of the essential mineral potassium. Nor will plastic surgery or the newer liposuction successfully eliminate cellulite deposits. Although surgery can be a very effective means of slicing away fat – if you can stand the pain, the expense and the possible complications afterwards – it does not ensure that none will ever return. In fact, if you have a toxic system, the cellulite will come back almost immediately, as you have not solved the problem. You may have cleared the drain for the time being, but you have not tackled the reason for its becoming blocked in the first place.

The anti-cellulite programme outlined in this book is not a treatment worked out by medical doctors. It has been developed over the years by nutritionists, aromatherapists and masseurs – and it is guaranteed to work.

There are no adverse side effects, no harsh drugs to take, and no dangers. If you have cellulite – and it is easy to check this by simple observation and pinching the thighs – then you owe it to yourself to get rid of it as quickly as possible.

After all, who wants a junk-laden system?

Chapter 3

The Anti-Cellulite Programme

Although cellulite has been regarded as a medical condition in France for many decades it was not until the early 1980s that a fully successful anti-cellulite regime began to be developed to help women rid themselves of unwanted and unattractive lumps and bumps.

As there were no clinical trials and no proper studies available on cellulite, the treatments were developed gradually, and by 'alternative' practitioners and therapists rather than doctors. As cellulite began to be understood it was realized that it would not go away permanently until the whole system could be cleaned both inside and out. Because although French doctors had been treating cellulite for many years, they did not understand what made it appear in the first place. They could offer treatment, but not prevention. Now it is possible to offer both.

The first alternative practitioners to provide a successful treatment for cellulite were aromatherapists, who used plant substances known as essential oils to help cleanse and detoxify the system. It was also realized that particular kinds of massage could help disperse lumps and bumps from problem areas.

However, it was not until a detoxifying diet was formulated that a completely successful anti-cellulite 'package' could be put together. The combination of the right diet, massage and the correct essential oils, means that cellulite can be completely eradicated, and the lumpy pockets of fat will disappear for ever.

The modern cellulite cure consists of four main elements: **Diet, Dry Skin Brushing, Aromatherapy and Massage**. All these four ingredients are absolutely essential in any effective anti-cellulite programme, but most vital is the diet. Because, even if you manage to get rid of some cellulite with oils and massage, it will always come back unless you can prevent more forming with the correct diet. The anti-cellulite diet does two main jobs: it cleanses and detoxifies the whole system to enable toxic wastes to be eliminated, and it prevents more cellulite from forming in the future.

THE DIET

When embarking on an anti-cellulite regime, it is essential to cleanse and detoxify the system from inside first. So you must begin with a very strict detoxifying diet.

The anti-cellulite diet now used by most therapists and masseurs grew out of research undertaken mainly in America, where it became apparent that very many of our modern illnesses were caused by large amounts of waste matter remaining in the body. Several American doctors began developing diets that could help people with a wide variety of serious illnesses, such as cancer, schizophrenia, arthritis, allergies and heart disease. One of the first of these doctors was Max Gerson, who successfully cured many patients of cancer with his raw-food diet. Then doctors Nathan Pritikin and Carl Pfeiffer began treating heart patients and the mentally ill with diet and nutritional therapies instead of the surgical and drug treatments which had become standard.

Gradually, further studies and research showed that many of our modern illnesses were caused by eating the wrong kinds of foods which eventually set up serious imbalances in the body. Avant-garde doctors in America also began to realize that much illness was caused by faulty elimination and by waste material staying in the system perhaps for years on end. Once the system is clogged up, they argued, the best method of treatment is to unclog it naturally, rather than rely on harsh drugs and purgatives.

These doctors understood that diuretics and laxatives could not be the answer, because as soon as you stopped taking the tablets the original problem would return and the body would start to clog up once more. In any case, many of the drugs had adverse side effects and would not lead to lasting health.

It seemed that what was needed above all was a diet which would help the body to eliminate its own long-held waste matter and encourage the lymphatic system, which transports wastes to eliminative organs, to do its job properly.

The theory was that a natural, wholefood diet would gradually enable the body to rid itself of accumulated undigested rubbish through the liver, kidneys, colon and skin.

It had been well known for several years that one of the reasons for faulty elimination of wastes was that certain foods tended to stay for too long in the system. If foods are not eliminated quickly then they tend to putrefy long before being expelled through the colon. Foods which would aid elimination, therefore, were those which had a quick 'transit time' – that is, they would pass through the entire alimentary tract before they had time to start decomposing.

And the foods which had the quickest transit times were those closest to nature – raw fruits and vegetables. Also, it was found that the quicker the transit time, the better the digestion, and the greater the likelihood of all the nutrients being absorbed.

Food tends to putrefy inside the body just as quickly as it does when left outside the fridge. If you leave fruit and vegetables outside the fridge it is usually several days before they start to go off. Milk left outside the fridge goes off extremely quickly, and meat will start to spoil in less than a day. Exactly the same thing happens inside the body. As the temperature inside the body is around 98.4°F, putrefaction of food takes place far more quickly than at normal room temperature.

The fresher and more natural the food, the more likely it is that it will pass through the body without undergoing any putrefaction whatever. One of the original formulators of the detoxifying diet, American doctor Robert Gray, found that when he ate a hundred per cent raw-food diet his stools lost all of their putrefactive odour and began to smell of whatever fruit he had been eating.

He also came to realize, by studying autopsies, that milk and dairy produce slowed down transit time by forming mucus, a sticky substance which could stick to the walls of the digestive tract and hinder transit time. Dr Gray, and other nutritional experts in America such as Dr Carl Pfeiffer and Nathan Pritikin, began to develop a diet which would help the whole body to cleanse and detoxify itself. This diet consisted mainly of fresh fruits and vegetables, eaten raw whenever possible, and a certain amount of fibre to aid digestion and effective elimination.

Dr Robert Gray was interested above all in cleaning the colon, and developed a diet which would enable accumulated waste matter to be eliminated. He understood that genuine health is impossible if the colon is impacted with old waste material it can no longer get rid of. His book, *The Colon Health Handbook*, explains how colons gradually become more and more impacted with waste material, mainly because we eat foods which encourage rubbish to stay in the system rather than being properly eliminated. In pre-literate societies, where only natural foods are eaten, many diseases associated with modern living simply do not exist.

Dr Gray realized that one of the most important aspects of a clean system is to have a properly working lymphatic system. There are two types of fluid designed to carry body wastes away – the lymph and the blood. Lymph is similar to blood except that it contains no red blood cells. Lymph vessels are contained in every cell in the body, and their job is to collect waste matter and eventually empty it back into the blood stream. The lymph vessels contain one-way valves and are composed of muscle tissue which pumps the lymph through these valves. When it is all working properly, wastes are taken away automatically via this system. When the lymph vessels are sluggish, however, wastes stay and accumulate in body cells. This is basically what happens when cellulite collects.

In its normal state, lymph is a colourless, watery fluid. Whenever there is over-accumulation of sticky mucoid matter, the lymphatic system is unable to remove it, and the result is congestion. So the very first step in getting rid of waste matter which has accumulated in body cells is to cleanse the lymphatic system, and allow excess toxic and mucoid material to drain away.

The best way to cleanse the lymphatic system is to go on a diet which excludes, as far as possible, foods which form mucus and clog up the body cells. Mucus-forming foods are basically dairy produce and fatty meats. Good lymph-clearing foods are fresh fruit and vegetables, organic if possible, wholegrains such as brown rice and millet, wheatbran and oatbran, lots of mineral water and only the occasional fish, eggs and lean meat. You should also avoid as far as possible alcohol, coffee, tea and cigarettes, substituting them with herb teas and fruit juices.

When therapists offering anti-cellulite treatments read Dr Gray's *The Colon Health Handbook* they instantly applied the principles to the cellulite problem. Clogged-up colons and waterlogged fatty cells are both manifestations of a related problem: failure to eliminate waste material.

The anti-cellulite diet is not a slimming diet in the usual sense. Although you will very probably lose weight while on it that is not its main purpose. The diet is not designed to get rid of ordinary fat so much as to encourage long-held body wastes to disperse. It helps to regard the anti-cellulite eating regime as, above all, a potent method of cleansing the system. The anti-cellulite diet is described in detail in the following chapter but, briefly, it consists of eating only fresh, natural foods and proteins. Normally on an anti-cellulite programme you will be asked to follow a fruit-and-mineral-water-only diet for a few days, to abstain from coffee, alcohol and tea, and to eat no meat or processed foods. After a week or so, the diet can be modified to some extent, but it is important to follow it fairly rigidly if you really want to be free of cellulite.

Remember also to drink at least one litre of plain water a day. If you find it difficult, as many people do at first, try to get into the habit of having a big glass of water by your side all day long. This is especially important if you work in a modern office. Drink a glass of water before you go to bed, and drink a glass first thing in the morning, before you have anything else to drink. As buying water can become expensive, try drinking plain boiled cooled water. If you can drink it warm, it is kinder to the system than ice-cold water, as well.

DRY SKIN BRUSHING

This is also extremely important, as it further helps clearing and cleansing of the lymphatic system. Dry skin brushing is probably an ancient technique, but it was revived in America in the early 1980s when colon-cleansing became all the rage. According to Dr Robert Gray, who recommended body brushing as well as a pure, natural diet for ensuring colon health, skin brushing is a 'highly effective technique for stimulating the expulsion of fresh mucoid material, hardened particulates or impacted mucoid matter, and other obstructions of the lymphatic system. Like the colon, the lymphatic system can contain stagnant accumulations of old waste matter.'

According to Robert Gray, you know when skin brushing is effective because you will begin to see lymph mucoid in the stools.

You have to use the right kind of brush. An ordinary loofah or bath mitt won't do, nor will those patent self-massagers advertised at high prices. There is only one kind of brush which does an effective job of helping to cleanse the lymphatic system, and that is a long-handled wooden brush made from natural fibres. At first, this kind of brushing will feel strange and unnatural but most people find that they enjoy it once they have become used to the sensation.

You have to begin body brushing at the same time as starting the diet. The two together will work wonders to get rid of cellulite that has been long held in body cells, and will encourage it to disperse. But as cellulite is often very hard to get rid of you may well need the help of aromatherapy and massage as well.

AROMATHERAPY

Most aromatherapists now offer anti-cellulite treatments. The essential oils used in aromatherapy work in conjunction with the diet and the body brushing to enable waste matter to empty itself into the lymphatic system.

Recent research on essential oils has established that many have a definite therapeutic effect, and that they do make a difference. For many years, aromatherapy was regarded as a 'French load of old cobblers' in much the same way as cellulite itself was (and still is in many circles), but it is rapidly becoming one of the most popular of all complementary therapies. One of the reasons for this is that people are now learning for themselves that it works.

We know now that aromatherapy oils are not just nice scents, but can be very potent remedies for a variety of ailments. There are specific oils for cleansing, detoxifying and stimulating circulation, and all of these will be used by a qualified aromatherapist to help bring about the body changes which will lead to loss of cellulite.

The use of aromatherapy oils to banish cellulite is explained fully in Chapter Six.

MASSAGE

This is also extremely important. Like aromatherapy, massage was for many years regarded as simply a beauty treatment indulged in by the idle rich. It has also had a rather unfortunate association with sleazy sex parlours. Now it is known that the right kind of massage can have a dramatic effect on the body. The type most often used in anti-cellulite treatments is known as **lymphatic drainage massage**. This is a very hard, tough kind of massage which pummels and kneads away at the cellulite deposits at the same time as activating the lymph nodes.

If you go for professional anti-cellulite treatments you will find that aromatherapy and massage are always used in conjunction with each other.

Note: There is a type of massage known as manual lymph massage, or MLD, which is used for cancer patients and which does not use essential oils. This is not the type of massage we are talking about. Anti-cellulite massage concentrates on the below-waist areas, although some therapists may activate lymph nodes in the neck as part of their treatment.

EXERCISE

This is an optional extra in any cellulite-banishing regime. Exercise can be very effective once you have managed to get rid of the worst of the cellulite and need to tone up the muscles. But there is not much point in embarking on rigorous exercise programmes while you have large areas of cellulite on your thighs. Although the condition is partly caused by a sedentary lifestyle, vigorous exercise will not make the slightest bit of difference to cellulite deposits that are already there.

In fact, many forms of exercise could make it worse, particularly anything that includes jumping up and down or pounding, such as jogging, jazz dancing, aerobics or California stretch-type exercises. These are emphatically NOT recommended for cellulite removal. They tend to put extra pressure on the joints and encourage the cellulite to harden and become even more impacted.

The best type of exercise is that which is both gentle and brisk at the same time, such as walking or swimming. Swimming is, in fact, excellent for cellulite sufferers as it exercises the legs without putting any undue strain on the joints.

Very often, women who have been on a rigorous anti-cellulite programme find that their legs become flabby and lacking in tone. This is often a temporary condition and can be likened to when you have just had a baby. The minute the baby is born, your stomach is flabby and stretched, like an empty sack. But after a very few weeks it tightens back up again and becomes flat, especially if you do the right kind of exercises to help yourself get back into shape.

Exactly the same process happens with cellulite removal. If the cellulite has been there for a very long time it will leave a certain amount of flab when it finally goes. Because once cellulite starts to disperse everything can happen very quickly – far too quickly for the skin to stay tight. Before long, though, the skin will start to 'fit' of its own accord. The time to embark on exercise is once the worst of the cellulite has gone.

RELAXATION AND DEEP BREATHING

Like most nasty things in life, cellulite is made worse by high levels of stress and anxiety, which release extra adrenalin into the system and make the liver work extra hard to try and get rid of the excess.

You should practise deep breathing whenever you have the opportunity, such as when relaxing in the bath. You do it like this: put both hands on your stomach and as you breathe in, inflate the abdomen. Breathe out slowly, letting the abdomen go back in. Repeat this whenever you think of it. This helps more oxygen to get into the system, and improves circulation.

CAN I GET RID OF CELLULITE BY MYSELF?

The answer to this is yes.

When I decided that I would try and get rid of my own cellulite I immediately booked up several treatments with a therapist who had been trained in lymphatic drainage massage as well as aromatherapy. I decided to enlist the help of a professional because I wanted to see for myself whether the treatments would work, and I was unsure that I would have the motivation all by myself. But it is perfectly possible to rid yourself of cellulite with the complete self-help programme which is outlined in this book.

The advantages of going to a therapist are that you have an objective assessment of your cellulite and your progress is monitored regularly. There is less chance that you will backslide and start drinking huge amounts of coffee or alcohol, or stuff yourself with cream cakes. Also, you can be sure that the right kind of oils will be used and the correct type of massage employed.

The decision whether to book up professional treatments or do it yourself depends on several factors – your pocket, your levels of self-motivation, the availability of trained therapists and the extent of your cellulite.

If you are young – still in your twenties – and have not therefore been a cellulite sufferer for very long, it is relatively easy to get rid of it by yourself. If, though, you are older, and have large amounts of cellulite which have been there for many years, you may find that professional help is invaluable.

When booking up a therapist it is vital that you go to somebody who really knows what she is doing. Unfortunately, as with all branches of alternative medicine, there is nothing to stop anybody setting up as an aromatherapist and charging high prices for doing precisely nothing. Names and addresses of reputable organizations are given on p.328.

Those who are not certain whether or not they have cellulite, or whether their problem is simply one of overweight, might find it useful to check with a trained therapist first. A good practitioner will give an honest answer. Do not assume that because you are over-weight or have thick thighs that you necessarily have cellulite. Your thick thighs may be simply a genetic inheritance. It's the lumpiness which indicates cellulite deposits, rather than actual girth. Cellulite has a distinctive appearance and must not be confused with ordinary flab or muscle. The orange-peel test is perhaps the most accurate one, although the cold feel and the tendency of the flesh not to go down immediately when pinched are other indications.

The other point about going to a professional is that you will be asked questions about high blood pressure, varicose veins or any other conditions which could be affected by the essential oils. If these do not apply to you, then of course there is no need to worry. But as a general precaution, any cellulite sufferer who also has other health problems, such as fluid retention, arthritis, high blood pressure, a heart condition, or any other serious illness, would be advised to seek professional help.

Usually, though, cellulite is a condition which is unaccompanied by any other illness. Most cellulite victims feel perfectly well and healthy, and have no idea that their bodies may be loaded down with toxic material.

DO PATENT ANTI-CELLULITE TREATMENTS WORK?

In a word, no. There is no cream or oil on the market which will magically melt away cellulite, nor is there likely to be. Most chemists' shops and department-store beauty counters are full of creams and lotions which purport to firm up flabby areas and improve body contours. Don't fall for them, especially as some of the ones on the market these days cost £20 or more for a small jar. Whatever cream, oil or lotion you buy, you will be wasting your money completely *unless* you are also prepared to go on the diet and undertake daily body brushing.

Remember that with any anti-cellulite programme, even if you go to a clinic which specializes in anti-cellulite treatments, 60 per cent of the work has to come from you.

Professor Sam Shuster, who is convinced that cellulite is a load of cobblers, does not believe that there is any cream on the market which can get rid of fat. He said in an interview with Maggie Drummond in *The Sunday Times*, June 1988, that any skin cream which got far enough down to have an effect on the body would have to be classed as a drug rather than a cosmetic, and would not be on general sale. These creams can do no more than a brisk walk, a body brush, or a quick rub-down with a loofah after a bath would do.

There are now very many aromatherapy-based anti-cellulite oils available. Beware of any which do not come in small dark glass bottles – essentials oils should *never* be in plastic containers – and always look for the word 'organic'. Some oils on sale have very few active ingredients, and you could be making an expensive mistake. Bodytreats, a specialist aromatherapy company, Daniele Ryman, Tisserand and Neals' Yard products are all the real thing.

These oils should always be used in conjunction with the programme outlined above, not just by themselves. But they are not, like many of the creams from major cosmetic houses, an expensive waste of money. They can work, but only together with the other treatments, and only if you apply them regularly and properly – there's nothing, unfortunately, which will make cellulite go away without hard work from you. This applies even if you decide to put your thighs into the care of a professional therapist.

In the end, there's only one person who can make the cellulite disappear, and that's you.

HOW DO I EMBARK ON AN ANTI-CELLULITE PROGRAMME?

The best way is gradually. Although the programme is extremely beneficial to health generally, it has to be realized that a toxic body takes time to heal itself. The more toxic the system is, the longer any cleansing programme will take.

Also, the body may react unfavourably at first to a drastic change in diet, however healthy this may be. We are primarily creatures of habit, and our bodies get used to whatever foods and drinks we give them. They may rebel when anything is withdrawn suddenly.

If you smoke, drink a lot of alcohol, eat junk foods, down several cups of coffee a day, and are also extremely sedentary it is unrealistic to suppose that you can revert to good habits in a single day. You will not be able to give up all your props and addictions at once, as this will represent too drastic a change for your system to handle. Also, you may well feel extremely deprived, and as if life is not worth living. It is only when people become released from their addictions and cravings that they come to realize that life is actually *more* enjoyable without the artificial props.

Those who smoke should make giving up or cutting down an urgent priority, long before they embark on the anti-cellulite regime. The difficulty of giving up smoking should never be underestimated. On the other hand, there is little point in undertaking the diet and the body brushing if you continue to smoke twenty or more cigarettes a day.

Once you have successfully conquered smoking, the next priority is to try to give up coffee and tea. Again, these beverages can form potent addictions, and be extremely hard to renounce. As one who has tried to give up both cigarettes and caffeine – though not at the same time – I can say that caffeine is definitely easier than nicotine. Nicotine is one of the most addictive drugs available – and one of the hardest to get out of the system.

Once you have managed to give up smoking, tea and coffee, then it will be time to embark on the anti-cellulite diet. This has to be very strict for two weeks, after which time it can be modified. You can even have the occasional cup of tea and coffee.

Once you start the diet you can consider that you have started the anti-cellulite regime proper. At the same time as beginning the diet, do the body brushing, the massage and the rubbing-in of essential oils.

You will find that after a very short time you will feel quite different about yourself. The first effect you will notice is that you go to the lavatory far more. You may also find that your skin breaks out in acne, that you get more earwax, and that your skin becomes very dry. You will probably also discover that you sweat more. These are all signs that the regime is working.

Those with extremely toxic systems may find themselves feeling rather unwell for three or four days. They may experience headaches, nausea, a sensation of disorientation, mood swings. All these will pass in about a week, at most.

HOW LONG BEFORE THE CELLULITE STARTS TO GO?

This depends on how strict you are with yourself and how much cellulite you have in the first place.

Most therapists reckon that six of their treatments – if possible two a week – combined with diet and brushing at home, will rid thighs of cellulite. In my own case it took far longer, but then I had suffered a severe cellulite problem for two decades.

Patricia Davis says she has rarely met anybody who needs more than ten treatments. You will almost certainly find that the cellulite starts to go after two weeks of the regime although of course we are all different.

Before starting, measure your thighs at the thickest part, and note down the measurement. Then, as you proceed with the programme, measure your thighs weekly, to see if there is any difference. There will certainly be a measurable loss after about a month.

If, after two weeks, you don't seem to be getting anywhere, don't give up hope. There is no cellulite in the world that can withstand the regime detailed in this book – so long as you follow it conscientiously and regularly. It is the *regularity of the treatments which does the trick. Nothing will work if it is remembered only occasionally.*

ANTI-CELLULITE PROGRAMME

PRE-PROGRAMME

PROGRAMME

Cut Out   *Cut Down*
Smoking   Alcohol
         Coffee

Take Up
Detoxifying diet for
   two weeks
Dry skin brushing daily
   before bath
Massage using
aromatherapy oils
after bath

POST-PROGRAMME

Keep Up
Exercise for toning
Healthy diet
Skin brushing twice a week
Occasional massage

Chapter 4

The Anti-Cellulite Diet: An Introduction

All restricted food-intake diets are tough, and the anti-cellulite diet is no exception. But for anybody who really wants to get rid of the lumps and bumps it's not an optional extra but an absolute necessity.

So many of us imagine that it would be really lovely to be able to eat and drink exactly what we like and not get fat, unhealthy, suffer from hangovers or develop cellulite. Unfortunately, the foods that we come to love and crave are often those that the body least wants, and finds hardest to digest.

So there's nothing for it but to make up your mind to become spartan and abstemious, at least until the cellulite has gone – and even afterwards, if you want it to stay away. Because like household dust, mice, greenfly on roses and ants, cellulite is always threatening to come back, and will do so at the very least opportunity.

I found that the best way to brainwash myself into sticking to the diet was to see myself as an ill person for whom the diet was a sure way to start getting better. It always helps if you can have a positive attitude, as that is what keeps you going, in the end.

The diet advocated here is the one first developed by Dr Weston Price, a dentist who went round the world recording the diet of people in pre-literate societies. He discovered time and again that the closer to nature their food, the healthier they stayed. The 'primitive' diets eaten by these people appeared to be the real key to their continuing good health. From this Dr Price concluded that the more removed from nature a diet was, the worse the general health of any community became. The more people ate white bread, chips, salted peanuts, crisps, and processed foods, the more they suffered from ill-health.

Over the years, Dr Price's ideas were taken up by other doctors and nutritionists who, until the 1980s, remained mainly on the fringes and were considered extremely cranky and peculiar. It wasn't until people such as health writer Leslie Kenton, nutritionists Celia Wright and Patrick Holford, and Dr Alan Stewart of the British Society for Nutritional Medicine, began writing about these diets in popular magazines that they gained general acceptance.

I say 'acceptance' but of course, the 'healthy' diet still is not accepted by everybody as the main ingredient of lasting health. Some authorities still laugh at the idea of 'detoxifying' and clearing the system of poisons by a pure diet. But the monastic, detoxifying diet is what health farms all over the world have been advocating for the past hundred years at least. Health farms were originally set up for the purpose of detoxifying over-indulgent Victorians whose lavish, eight-course meals laden with fats and meats had led to obesity and a number of degenerative diseases.

It is only since the mid-1970s that the natural detoxifying diet has been put forward as the best way to start getting rid of cellulite. Now it has been eagerly adopted by all therapists who treat these lumps and bumps, and their grateful clients know that they owe their newly cellulite-free limbs in large part to following the recommended diet.

The first step in any cellulite-removing regime is a thorough cleansing of the system. The more clogged up the body is, the more drastic the cleansing will have to be. If it is really bad you may do well to eat nothing but fruit and vegetables, raw whenever possible, for about two weeks. This gives the liver and lymphatic system a chance to unclog and to start working efficiently once more to expel the accumulated wastes. When eating a fruit-only diet, you should stick to one variety at each meal. That is, only bananas, only grapes, or only apples, for example. The reason for this is that different fruits have different acid levels and may interfere with each other.

As mentioned in the previous chapter, you really have to cut out tea and coffee, ideally drinking neither for at least two weeks. Now, very many people find that cutting out tea and coffee is quite the hardest part of the diet. This is because over the years they have become addicted to them, usually quite without realizing it.

Coffee, as we have seen, is a potent cellulite-causer, and the same goes for all caffeine-loaded drinks – tea, chocolate, colas – even the calorie-free variety. Don't drink these either while you are trying to rid yourself of cellulite.

When attempting to cut out tea and coffee you will soon know if you are addicted. Try going without either of them for forty-eight hours, and see how you feel when drinking herbal substitutes instead. If you are used to drinking more than three cups of tea or coffee in a single day you will most probably experience quite severe withdrawal symptoms. These, say many doctors, can be quite as bad as withdrawing from heroin.

Caffeine is a potent drug, and its sudden withdrawal temporarily upsets the system, causing very bad migraine headaches and a feeling of disorientation. In my case the migraine I suffered from sudden caffeine withdrawal was so bad that I had to go to bed. I simply couldn't work. In addition, I felt miserable and depressed. Assured that these symptoms would pass in time, I waited and waited. It took about a week for the worst of the symptoms to wear off, but I never really felt well while not drinking any tea or coffee.

In the end, my therapist sympathized and advised me to go back to one cup of real coffee a day, so long as it was made with freshly ground beans that were kept in the freezer to ensure freshness. I did, and instantly my spirits lifted. Now I drink just that one delicious, not-to-be-missed cup of coffee a day, and have one cup of Luaka or ordinary tea in the afternoon. But on an anti-cellulite regime the coffee you drink must be real, made from freshly ground beans. You should not under any circumstances drink the instant variety, as this not only has caffeine added but is made by a high-tech process which renders it completely artificial.

At the same time as cutting down on tea or coffee, it is important to increase considerably your intake of mineral water. Any mineral water on the market will do, but try not to drink tap water too much. When starting the cleansing regime, you should drink as many as eight glasses of mineral water a day, if you can remember to do so. In my case, I found constant Perrier and Badoit so boring that I kept forgetting to drink them. For me, the carbonated drinks are slightly more interesting and fun to drink than the still ones, although not much. Some people have said that they can get 'high' on Perrier, and there is at least one recent study to show that if people believe they are drinking alcohol when they are not, they can still get tipsy.

While on the subject of getting tipsy, it is important to avoid all alcohol, if possible, when on the initial cleansing programme. Alcohol has a similar effect on body metabolism to caffeine, in that it raises blood sugar content instantly, and then the body has to work hard to accommodate the extra glucose. As with caffeine, it tends to end up in fat stores eventually. Also, taking alcohol whilst on a cleansing diet tends to overload the liver, which is now having to work over-time anyway to eliminate all the waste matter rapidly being freed from cellulite-loaded areas.

Fruit juices can be drunk in moderation, and prefer-ably diluted with mineral water, as 'neat' they can be too strong for a system in the process of detoxification. Look out for the natural brands, such as Copella or Aspall, which are made with real fruits instead of concentrates. Of course, avoid all sugar-laden fruit drinks and squashes.

Now we come on to the thorny subject of food. Ide-ally, all your food should be raw, organically grown, eaten the day of purchase, or picked from your own garden, unfrozen, unprocessed, unsalted, untreated in any way. Clearly, this kind of diet is virtually impossi-ble for anybody to follow at home, although some health farms specialize in this kind of therapy.

While on the cleansing regime it is also more or less impossible to eat in a restaurant, go out to dinner, or have a quick snack in a café. You have to make up your mind to be an unsociable hermit, so it is best to pick a fortnight when you have few social or work engagements. It may seem hard, and the ultimate in deprivation, but if you keep reminding yourself that the whole purpose of the cleansing regime is to give the cellulite deposits a reasonable chance of dis-persing, you will be encouraged to continue.

Some people with really bad cellulite are put on a fruit juice fast for a few days, to ensure that the worst of the toxins are eliminated quickly. I found I could not exist on the fast, because I was too busy and active all the time. Most diet books which advocate fasting advise you to pick days when you are not doing much more than mooching around at home. But very few of us in reality have days like that. It is a good idea, though, at least to try to eat nothing but fruit and vegetables for that important two weeks. The main idea behind the fruit-and-vegetable-only diet is that these are the foods the body finds easiest to digest. They will not put any kind of strain on the liver or kidneys. The more difficult foods are to digest, the less chance you will have of the cellulite disappearing. You can't expect the organs of elimination to be able to do everything at once. Anything processed, cooked or generally denatured adds to the burden on the digestive system.

Some people allege that they feel wonderful straight-away on an all-fruit-and-vegetable diet. Many more will feel quite terrible at first. This is mainly because the body takes time to adapt to any radical change of diet. This applies even if you are changing from an unhealthy to an extremely healthy diet. So you should be prepared for some feelings of disorientation and discomfort, for cravings, depression and bad temper, at first. These are all withdrawal symptoms, a sign that something is happening, and they won't last for more than a few days.

Another reason why an all-plant-food diet can cause initial problems is that we tend to underestimate the sheer force of habit. Many people embarking on a stringent diet for the first time simply are not prepared for the drastic body changes that might happen. You will certainly find changes in bowel movements and frequency of urination. You may also find that you sweat more, and may erupt in the kind of spots you haven't had since adolescence. Some women also experience menstrual changes.

In my case I found that initially, apart from headaches, I suffered from insomnia, which is unusual for me. Not only that, but my nights were disturbed by visions of wonderful toast dripping with butter, cups of coffee, meals in restaurants and so on. In his searing book on concentration camps, *If This is a Man*, Primo Levi writes about how the inmates used to dream about food night after night. Something similar may happen when you first embark on an all-fruit-and-vegetable diet. If it does, it's just withdrawal symptoms, not a sign that you are chronically mal-nourished, as the concentration camp victims were. You may also feel rather miserable for no apparent reason, and this is again a sign that you are suffering from withdrawal. Don't forget that butter, cream, bread and cakes can be quite as addictive as any drugs – and sudden deprivation may have a marked effect.

None of these symptoms is anything to worry about; they are simply indications that the body is at last getting rid of toxic wastes. To add insult to injury, it is extremely unlikely that you will notice any difference in the cellulite at first. It will usually be a week or two before the stuff even begins to shift.

Although the initial cleansing diet consists of fruit and vegetables, don't imagine that any old fruit and veg will do. Far from it. Even here, you have to be careful. Citrus fruits such as oranges and grapefruit are out except very occasionally, as they are rather rough on the liver. But definitely in are bananas, apples, pears, pineapple, all the exotica such as mangoes, papaya, passion fruit, sharon fruit (the hard, orange-coloured fruits which come from Israel), kiwi fruit, grapes, strawberries (very good – especially English ones), raspberries, blackberries. If you are eating fruit alone for the first few days you can eat almost any amount – up to six pounds a day. You should eat some fruit every two hours, otherwise you will start to feel hungry, and should drink plenty of mineral water in between. Most nutritional experts do not advise eating and drinking together, as water dilutes the digestive juices.

Good vegetables are: potatoes, spinach, cauliflower, broccoli, cabbage, mangetout, beans, turnips, swedes, green peppers, carrots, celery. Not all of these can be eaten raw, of course, but wherever possible, eat without cooking. Spinach, cauliflower and broccoli are delicious raw, with a small amount of vinaigrette or lemon dressing. Again, the portions of raw vegetables can be as large as you like.

People who are not used to eating like this, or who have never been to a health farm where this kind of diet is standard, will find it very peculiar. Do try to persevere, though, as it will really get the cellulite shifting when combined with body-brushing and the other treatments.

Here is a typical day's eating and drinking plan for the first two weeks on an anti-cellulite regime:

ON RISING

A glass of hot water with a small amount of lemon, or one of the 'wake-up' herb teas such as Early Morn, or a glass of cold water. Always use mineral rather than tap water for early morning drinks if you can.

BREAKFAST

A couple of bananas, apples, or a huge bunch of grapes. That's it. Plus, of course, mineral water either half an hour before or half an hour after the fruit.

Those who know that they are simply not going to be able to manage on fruit alone should not reach for the nearest slice of bread, but should nibble sunflower, sesame or pumpkin seeds. If you have a coffee grinder, grind up equal amounts of these seeds and sprinkle them on the fruit. Then you won't feel hungry, although it may be difficult at first not to eat that really delicious toast, butter and marmalade that the others are tucking into.

MID MORNING

Eat more fruit if you are at home. If at work, take a selection of fruit and seeds with you. Bananas are particularly good at assuaging hunger.

LUNCH

Whenever possible, eat a large salad consisting of raw vegetables. Carrots, cauliflower and broccoli are all quite filling, and you can eat as much of them as you like. Those who are not used to raw vegetables may find eating them very odd at first, although they are becoming more accepted nowadays. If you can't be bothered to cut and chop your own, most supermarkets do some wonderful ready-prepared salads which come complete with dressings. Although these bought salads may seem expensive, they can actually work out cheaper than buying whole cauliflowers, pounds of carrots, broccoli, etc, which you may have a job to finish before they start going off.

You can now buy juicers, which are well worth the outlay, to have fresh fruit and vegetable juices throughout the day. Also, look for seasonal selections of organic vegetables, now on sale in all supermarkets. Beetroot is a good blood cleanser, and has the added advantage of enabling you to monitor your motions. Urine will be slightly pinky-coloured, and faeces will have a pinkish tinge about them too, to enable you to time transit times. As a general rule, the quicker the transit time the better. It should be about 36 hours.

A new non-wheat brand of pasta, Organum, is available in many shops. Also look for Chinese noodles made of rice. If you are avoiding dairy products, it is a good idea to take a calcium supplement. Higher Nature (details at end of book) have a particularly potent one.

MID-AFTERNOON

Have a cup of herb tea if you are feeling like crawling up the wall by now, and some more fruit. Throughout the day, drink lots of mineral water, but not too many herb teas. Some of them can be quite strong.

SUPPER

Here you can have some vegetable soup, sprinkled with ground seeds, and then another huge vegetable salad, or just some more fruit if you can manage it.

BEFORE BED

You'll be sick to death of fruit and vegetables by now, and anyway they don't seem to be very good last thing at night. If you really feel you must have something before retiring, have an oatcake, or an organic rice cake thinly covered with sesame seed spread. As a bedtime drink you can try Barleycup. Some people like this drink but I could never get used to it. If you haven't had too many cups of herb tea throughout the day, have one now, formulated for late at night. An 'early-morning' herb tea at this time may keep you awake.

Note: When embarking on this diet, you may find it difficult to get to sleep. This is partly because you are changing your eating habits radically and your body has not adjusted to them, and partly because you are feeling deprived of tea and coffee. A bedtime herb drink will help you get over insomnia which in any case should not last for too long. It all depends on how poisoned your system is and for how long you have been eating a denatured diet.

Those who find this diet impossible should cook a large quantity of brown rice and keep it in the fridge to turn to when, and if, hunger becomes acute and painful. Actually, the problems don't lie so much with actual hunger as with the fact that you are not now eating any of the comforting foods.

When starting the anti-cellulite diet you have to give priority to this form of eating. It is not a good idea to do it at the same time as moving house, starting a new job, or undergoing any emotional or physical upheavals. Getting rid of the cellulite is hard work and upheaval enough, and you should, ideally, concentrate on this task alone for a time.

After ten days to two weeks you can introduce a wider variety of foods to your diet. You can start off in the morning with porridge or muesli, in both cases not made with milk. Muesli can be soaked overnight in a little mineral water or fruit juice and eaten with yogurt in the morning – so long as it's natural, low-fat, live yoghurt and not of the thick and creamy variety. You can eat oatcakes spread with sesame or sunflower seed paste, or a margarine such as Vitaquell. Tofu, a cheese-like substance made from soya flour, is a very good substitute for milk, cream and cheese and is a wonderfully adaptable food. And you can now have that most marvellous treat, a cup of real coffee every single day.

While on the regime, avoid all dairy products as much as possible. You can make nut 'cream' which is almost (although not quite) as good as double cream, from simply blending together cashew nuts or almonds, a little honey and enough water to give pouring consistency. Your best friend now is not diamonds, but a food processor. In fact, I would almost say that this gadget is essential for anybody on an anti-cellulite diet.

If you have the occasional lapse during the first two weeks' anti-cellulite diet, at least make sure that you have a big salad at every main meal. To some extent, this will neutralize the bad effect of anything else you might have eaten.

Two of the best kinds of food for anybody wishing to keep cellulite away for ever are nuts and pulses.

Those who are vegetarian or who have drastically reduced their meat and fish intake may worry about getting enough protein, although you do not have to worry about this until the initial two weeks are up – you'll have plenty of stored fats to keep you going. Nuts and pulses provide plenty of protein. At one time it was difficult to buy a variety of pulses but now lentils of all colours, soya beans, flageolets, blackeye beans, red and black kidney beans, mung beans and split peas are on sale at practically all supermarkets. You can also easily buy brazils, almonds and cashew nuts – all manna to the cellulite shifter.

Pulses and nuts are very versatile. You can put them into soups, stews, curries and salads, or make them into patés, and they will keep you feeling pleasantly full for hours. Pulses can be flavoured with fresh ginger and herbs and eaten with brown rice. As time goes on, you will experience new taste sensations. Many people who have been on a detoxifying and cleansing diet for any length of time find they simply can't go back to their old ways. Cakes, white pastry, thick cream and biscuits start to taste heavy and cloying. You can almost sense the cellulite going back on if you bite into one of these products.

Don't imagine, though, that you have to say good-bye to these foods for ever. The occasional slice of Black Forest gateau or dish swimming in cream sauce does you no harm at all, and if you find it absolutely delicious, it probably does you good psychologically, too. I remember in the thick of my own detoxifying diet I felt ravenous during the interval of a concert at the Royal Festival Hall. As usual, there was nothing I could eat and, in desperation, I had just one Cornetto. I can't remember when I've enjoyed anything quite so much. It was absolutely wonderful – but I didn't crave another Cornetto for months and months afterwards. That one little treat was enough.

It is a good idea to keep a food and drink diary at this stage to record exactly what you are eating, and to monitor good and bad reactions to food. You may discover that the days seem very long without tea or coffee, and particularly if you are used to drinking alcohol at every meal. You will almost certainly miss chocolate, cocoa, cream, cheese, bread and butter at first. Think of them not as delicious foods, but as poisons which all add to the cellulite load – then it will be easier to avoid them.

Until the cellulite goes, you should avoid all white flour and refined products. This goes for white rice, white pasta, all shop-bought cakes and biscuits, white bread and rolls. Instead, you can buy buckwheat spaghetti, wholemeal macaroni and other pasta, brown rice and wholemeal bread. Dried fruit can be eaten in moderation, and is best soaked overnight. You will probably find you become an aficionado of the local health food shop and, before very long, an expert on healthy foods.

Very attractive breakfasts and desserts can be made by blending together in a food processor soaked dried fruit such as hunza apricots, a small amount of natural yoghurt, a squeeze of lemon and real honey. Some honeys, particularly the ones that are the 'produce of several countries', are not the real thing at all, but highly processed. As one might expect, it is the more expensive honeys that are likely to be the best ones. As so little is eaten at one time, it is worth buying the better brands.

As a committed vegetarian myself, I naturally do not advocate eating fish and meat. I must say that vegetarianism *per se* made not the slightest difference to my cellulite. I did get thinner, but the cellulite stayed firmly in place, blast it. But for non-vegetarian cellulite removers, occasional fish or meat does no harm. Most fish, I understand, is not artificially fed and reared, but ideally you should avoid all meats which have been intensively farmed, such as turkey, chicken and pork. Lamb is usually all right, and is, in fact, one of the better meats you can get today. Beef is often full of antibiotics and should be eaten only occasionally. You can now buy additive-free meat – butchers who sell this advertise it as such.

Celia Wright, author of the excellent book *The Wright Diet*, which forms the basis for the anti-cellulite diet advocated by most therapists, strongly advises against eating pork in any form. She says that almost all pork is infected with a parasite called trichinosis, which is easily passed to humans. Also bacon, sausages, tinned, frozen and preserved meats should not be eaten by anybody serious about keeping cellulite off. All these products are likely to contain high amounts of salt, other preservatives, and artificial colours and are usually highly processed into the bargain. Those who have a cellulite problem should, ideally, avoid processed and artificial foods altogether for the rest of their lives. However, you should not try to give everything up at once. This is patently impossible.

The good news about alcohol is that, after the first booze-free fortnight of the serious anti-cellulite regime, you can gradually introduce the occasional drink back into your life. In fact, if you can drink only organic wines, they will even do you good. Wines with additives, such as sugar and chemicals, may not do the system any good, but the organic ones actually help digestion.

To sum up, you should avoid, at least for the first fortnight of anti-cellulite eating: bread and butter, milk and dairy products, meat and fish if possible, all processed foods, anything cooked, salted nuts and crisps, all preserved meats, spirits, smoked foods, instant coffee (best to avoid this at all times, anyway), and ready-frozen meals. All these substances are cellulite-forming and will undo all the good work you are doing in other areas.

Also best avoided are all products made with white or refined flour, bread, biscuits, ice-cream, pastry, bought sauces, pasta, and all fried foods.

One of the earliest signs that the cellulite is starting to go is that you urinate much more frequently. Indeed, as the system starts to shake itself up, you may find you are going to the toilet up to three times before breakfast. Also, on the fruit diet you will find a definite increase in bowel movements. This, too, indicates that cellulite is starting to shift.

Books such as Leslie and Susannah Kenton's *Raw Energy* and Celia Wright's *The Wright Diet* give more detailed information on eating the all-fruit-and-vegetable diet. If you can manage it for a whole two weeks then you will be well on the way towards shifting that awful cellulite. And, as a plus, your general health will improve by leaps and bounds as well.

Chapter 5

Dry Skin Brushing

I first came across the concept of dry skin brushing in Dr Robert Gray's *The Colon Health Handbook*, where he recommended five minutes' skin brushing a day in order to cleanse the lymphatic system and get it working efficiently once more.

Body brushing, he explained, is a very effective way of enabling the lymphatic system to clear itself and expel waste material which has been held for a long time inside the body. In addition this technique can correct inflammations of the lymph nodes. In order to be really effective, any skin brushing programme must be kept up for several months, and it is important to use a special kind of brush which has particularly hard and scratchy bristles.

When I first read that scouring yourself all over with a dry, scratchy brush could tone up the whole internal system I found it hard to believe. How could brushing yourself on the outside make any difference to what happened inside your body? Back brushes and loofahs have long been a standard part of bathroom

equipment, but the idea that the brushing could activate internal organs sounded very suspect indeed, just
one more of those crazy Californian notions which
were being put about in the early 1980s.

Of course, Robert Gray was only talking about the
power of skin brushing to help the colon to clear. His
book did not mention cellulite at all, and it was to be
several years before skin brushing was advocated for
cellulite removal. But not long after reading Robert
Gray's book, I began to hear more and more about the
benefits of dry skin brushing. A number of alternative
practitioners in Britain soon became extremely enthusiastic about it and were advising their patients to
brush themselves daily before having their bath, as it
was all wonderfully stimulating and would help you
feel alive and awake, as well as releasing new levels of
energy.

As time went on, enormous benefits were being
claimed for dry skin brushing. I don't know who
invented, or developed, the technique, but it rapidly
became extremely respectable among practitioners
of complementary therapies. Orthodox doctors, of
course, laughed it to scorn.

As soon as aromatherapists and other practitioners
who were trying to treat cellulite heard about the technique they felt certain it could be of enormous use in
getting rid of the toxins which cause the lumpy
deposits. They tried it out, and soon discovered that it
was just as effective in dispersing cellulite as it was

supposed to be in helping to cleanse the colon. As both conditions were caused, above all, by a sluggish lymphatic system, anything which could help one problem would almost certainly be efficacious for the other. Body brushing soon caught on because it was, above all, cheap and easy to do. It did not require expensive equipment, and anybody could learn how to do it very quickly.

Nowadays, enthusiasts are claiming that the technique has many benefits apart from its ability to remove cellulite or clean out colons. Skin brushing can tone up your whole system, encourage ordinary fat cells to disperse, invigorate the brain and also remove stress and tension from the system, according to its advocates. In a very few short years, body brushing has become a standard technique recommended by those doctors, nutritionists and healers who are interested in natural healing rather than relying on drugs, surgery and hospitals.

Another American expert, Dr Jack Soltanoff, author of *Natural Healing*, reckons that just five minutes' skin brushing a day can improve digestion, aid metabolism and impart new levels of energy – as well as get rid of cellulite. In his book he writes:

The technique is a mild form of acupressure and acupuncture performed without piercing the skin. The only tool that is required is a scrub or handbrush. When followed correctly and in the proper sequence, the dry friction skin bath has far-reaching beneficial effects on your health because it affects all the inner organs in the remote parts of your body via the reflexes of the nervous system.

As your skin and circulation are affected, the technique produces a wonderful feeling and a warm glow ... The dry skin friction bath is extremely beneficial for those whose office jobs force them to sit at a desk all day, and especially those who must sit in rigid or cramped positions in front of computer terminals or typewriters day after day.

Dr Soltanoff considers that the other eliminative organs, such as the bowels, lungs and kidneys, are abused daily by most of us with the overconsumption of 'refined, commercialized processed foods, tobaccos, coffee, tea, chocolate, alcohol'. The skin-brushing technique has the power, he says, to stimulate these organs into eliminating effectively.

On the ability of skin brushing to disperse cellulite, Dr Soltanoff writes:

This technique works on cellulite by gradually breaking down the obese liquid-filled fatty tissues and slowly releasing the toxic fluids through various channels, particularly the lymphatic system. With regular daily use, your legs will firm up and tighten. You'll have a much younger figure, and that in itself will make you feel terrific.

Skin brushing seems like a fairly passive activity, in that it can be carried out in your own bathroom, but some advocates believe that it can even replace jogging. A number of American natural-health experts are now saying that five minutes of the right kind of body brushing a day is as good as half an hour's pounding the streets. You don't get the aerobic effect of course, but the benefits to your circulation and digestive system are as great.

The technique can also retard the ageing process of the skin, greatly improve your figure, and even enable you to banish apathy and boredom, say some American practitioners. Dr Soltanoff is such an enthusiast for daily body brushing that he maintains it is possible literally to brush all your troubles away – mental, physical and even emotional ones.

Dr Soltanoff, a chiropractor who recommends the skin-brushing technique to all of his patients, believes along with Dr Robert Gray that there is no better way of activating and cleansing the lymphatic system. The skin, he says, is the largest eliminative organ in the body and when it doesn't function properly, an enormous burden is placed on all other eliminative organs, such as the bowels, lungs and kidneys. They have to work far harder than they should. In an average day, says Dr Soltanoff, the skin will eliminate as much waste matter as the kidneys or lungs. The trouble is that for most of us the skin has become clogged up too, and is less efficient as an organ of elimination than it ought to be because the pores cannot get rid of waste products properly. This means they stay in the system and add to the burden of waste material which eventually leads to cellulite and other problems caused by faulty elimination of rubbish.

Kitty Campion, a British herbalist who became converted to body brushing in the early 1980s, now uses it on many patients who go to her clinic near Stoke-on-Trent. 'When you first try it out,' she warns, 'skin brushing feels very strange and unusual. It's rather scratchy and uncomfortable, if you use the correct kind of brush, and is not at all the same sensation as brushing with a loofah, for instance. But though it seems so new, in fact the technique of skin brushing for health has been known for thousands of years. We are rediscovering it, rather than inventing something new. I find that most people wonder however they managed without it once they get used to it.'

Kitty Campion says that many people who come to her for herbal treatments are in very poor health, even if they are not always aware of this. 'A common condition these days is that the kidneys and lungs are not functioning as well as they should. They have become sluggish, and inefficient at eliminating waste material. I usually recommend skin brushing to all my clients, as a first step on their way back to health. It sounds odd to say that just by brushing, you can activate internal systems and get them working again, but that's exactly what happens.'

She lists the benefits of skin brushing in her book, *A Woman's Herbal*. Firstly, daily brushing removes the dead layers of skin and other impurities, allowing the pores to eliminate without obstruction. Secondly, the technique stimulates circulation, so that the blood nourishing those organs of the body which lie near the surface reaches them effectively. Thirdly, it is an excellent way of removing cellulite and clearing the lymphatic system.

The main benefit, though, according to Kitty Campion, is that it helps to prevent premature ageing and induces a wonderful sense of well-being. She writes: 'Many of my patients complain a lot about the things I ask them to do but I have never yet encountered one who has complained about skin scrubbing. Once they get used to it, they love it!'

If you want to see for yourself just how many dead cells fly off when skin brushing, says Kitty, brush in bright sunlight and you'll see huge amounts of dust coming off.

Frances Clifford, the aromatherapist who successfully helped me to get rid of two decades of cellulite deposits, is also extremely enthusiastic about dry skin brushing. She says, 'Body brushing is wonderful for sloughing off dead skin cells. It stimulates blood flow and gets oxygen to all parts of the body. The technique strengthens the immune system as well, and is extremely good for anybody suffering from low energy levels. I do skin brushing now on all my clients, and they love it, because it makes them feel so good.'

It was after investigating the benefits of dry skin brushing for myself that I bought a brush and gave the technique a try. I must say that I hated it at first. The brush was so very scratchy, and I could only apply very light pressure. Also, it hurt a lot when I stepped into the bath right after brushing my skin. But I persevered and soon got used to it. My skin started to welcome the daily brushing. After a few weeks, I started to enjoy it and then missed it if I didn't do it for any reason.

I now have no doubt whatever that skin brushing played a major part in enabling my own cellulite to disappear, and so I can heartily recommend the practice from personal experience. It can do you no possible harm, and will only do good, so long as you never break the skin when brushing.

It is essential to have the correct type of brush. This must be very hard, and made of natural, not synthetic fibres. A soft bristle brush won't have the same effect at all. Most body brushing experts recommend a long-handled brush made of Mexican cactus fibre. The handle should be detachable, and made of natural wood, with a strap across the brush.

These brushes are very stiff and scratchy when you first use them, and you may feel that they will take your skin off. If yours scratches too much, soak it for a few hours in the bathroom basin, then dry overnight in the airing cupboard. It will then be soft enough to use without harming the skin.

In order for dry skin brushing to be really effective, the strokes you apply have to be firm and long. Start with light pressure and gradually build up, as your skin becomes used to the sensation. You will discover in time that the skin can take quite hard pressure, but it will probably be tender at first.

Dry skin brushing in this way is not the same thing as rubbing your skin with a loofah, bath mitt or ordinary back brush. None of these will work to break down cellulite, or activate the lymphatic system because they go soft very quickly. It is only all-over brushing with the right kind of brush which will have this effect.

If you are interested only in brushing to get rid of cellulite, you can just concentrate on these areas. The pressure can be as hard as you like. Brush up the back of the leg in long, single strokes (see diagram). Then when you get to the thigh, brush upwards as

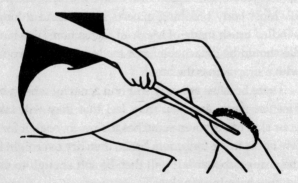

vigorously as you can where the cellulite is at its most dense. Finish off by brushing the buttocks equally hard, in any direction. Usually, skin brushing has to be done in the direction of the heart, but circular movements round the buttocks are best.

Brush both legs an equal amount and then get into the bath. You will find that the bath water makes your skin tingle pleasantly. If you are doing body brushing in conjunction with aromatherapy you should rub in the essential oils straight after you get out of the bath, again paying particular attention to the cellulite areas. The best time for applying the massage oils is after body brushing and a bath because then the pores will be open and unclogged. Kitty Campion advises a short, cold shower after a long, hot bath to maximize the effect of skin scrubbing, but not everybody will be able to stand the invigorating effect of this treatment. From a cellulite-removing point of view, there is no need to add the cold shower to the range of treatments.

If you find the brushing has left long scratches, or makes you look as though you had walked through a field of brambles, you are either doing it too hard or the brush needs more soaking. The brushing should never be allowed to break the skin. In any case, never brush over broken skin.

THE WHOLE-BODY BRUSH

You don't, of course, have to limit skin brushing to cellulite-dense areas. A whole-body brush will tone up the system even more, and increase the benefits.

This is how to do it.

You should start by brushing your fingers and hands. Hold your hand with fingers splayed, and brush between each finger a few times. Brush on top of the hand and then the palm, as many times as you like. Repeat this with the other hand.

Now do your arms. Brush in long strokes from the wrist to the elbow, then from the elbow to the shoulder. Always use long, firm, bold strokes, and remember always to brush in the direction of the heart.

After this, do your toes and feet. Put one leg on the rim of the bath or basin, and brush across the tops of the toes. Brush the soles of the feet, then around the ankles. Again, use the firmest possible strokes. Brush the leg up to the knee, going all round the leg and using long strokes from the ankle. Repeat this about fourteen times. Now brush the thighs and buttocks. Repeat with the other leg. As you brush, you will soon get to know the cellulite areas, and you will see them gradually diminishing over the weeks. But don't expect that one vigorous brushing session will send them away. For really bad cellulite, you may have to keep this practice up for several months. Anybody who wishes to stop the cellulite coming back – as it will always try to do – should build body brushing into their everyday lives.

After having a real good go at the worst areas of cellulite you should now move up to the neck. Brush downwards from the head, front and back. Now do the shoulders, this time brushing downwards, to keep in the direction of the heart.

Cellulite sufferers can help to activate the lymphatic system by holding the brush in the armpit and rotating it seven times to the left and seven times to the right. This action, if repeated daily, gets the lymph nodes working again. Women who visit an aromatherapist for the removal of cellulite will discover that the therapist always does this towards the end of a treatment.

Now do the front and sides of the body. Women should avoid brushing over the nipples, but can brush over the breasts, perhaps with lighter pressure. Some authorities do not advise brushing over the stomach and abdomen, as the action can be too strong. It is probably better to leave this area alone, and go on to the back. You will need the long handle to reach the back and again, long, firm strokes should be employed.

Although this procedure may sound complicated, in fact it is very simple indeed and takes no more than five minutes per session. Women with very bad cellulite should spend at least five minutes a day on body brushing for two months. After this length of time, the body gets used to the brushing and the technique is less effective. When this has happened, you should brush every other day. Kitty Campion says, 'The idea is to surprise your skin. Skin brushing is subject, as is the use of herbs, to homeostatic resistance – that is, your skin will get used to it and stop responding so well.' She suggests juggling the days of the week around, so that your skin does not always know when it is going to get the treatment. Other therapists I have spoken to confirm the fact that skin brushing loses its efficacy after a time, and that breaks have to be built into the treatment.

Some women find that once they start on a serious anti-cellulite regime they can't stop, and tend to over-do it at first. But the body has to be helped to get rid of its cellulite gently and safely, and you have to be patient. Just because five minutes of body brushing is good, it doesn't follow that ten minutes or quarter of an hour will be much better. Be gentle at first, and build up pressure gradually once your skin has got used to the sensation.

You may find that your skin does funny things when you embark on brushing it. Remember that this is not just a beauty treatment but an actual health-promoting regime. Most people find that their skin changes texture after a few weeks of brushing. In my case it went extremely dry for a time, and all the massage oils in the world didn't seem to make any difference. But after this, it seemed to go very smooth and unlined. Those who find that their skin seems to alter should just continue with the brushing. It can't do you any harm.

The technique is safe for everybody, except for those who have damaged, infected or broken skin. People who have eczema, psoriasis or any other skin complaint should not use the brush on affected areas. You can brush where the skin is free from damage, though the technique should also not be used on any areas where you have bad varicose veins.

Dry skin brushing is, of course, equally effective for men and women. Men who know they have sluggish kidneys or livers will definitely benefit from an all-over skin brush every morning. If done first thing in the morning it will give a wonderful wake-up sensation.

Some people have even found that dry skin brushing can actually help them to reverse quite serious illnesses. Val Harrod, a British Telecom officer from Stoke-on-Trent, had suffered from an undiagnosed and quite serious liver complaint for many years. She went to doctor after doctor but, although her hands and the soles of her feet were extremely yellow, nobody could discover what was wrong. In the end, worried because she often had to take time off work through illness, Val went to see herbalist Kitty Campion. She said: 'I went to Kitty because I could no longer believe what the doctors were telling me. Kitty diagnosed my condition through iridology (where general health is assessed by the condition of the eyes) and said my liver and lymphatic system were almost completely clogged up. Instead of getting rid of waste, I was just retaining it.

'She recommended skin brushing, and showed me how to do it. Of course, I was extremely sceptical at first, but I tried it, and gradually my liver started to clear. The yellowness on my hands and feet disappeared, and my eyes became brighter. My skin became more alive and the waste started to disperse. Now that I realize how effective skin brushing can be I shall certainly do it for the rest of my life. I do have a faulty liver, which will never work properly and will always be liable to clog up. But I know now that regular skin brushing can prevent the problem from building up.'

Val carries out skin brushing every other day for about ten minutes, and says: 'If you've never done skin brushing before, you can get quite a fright as you see the scales coming off your skin in huge amounts. It makes you realize just how clogged up your pores can get. For me, skin brushing doesn't just have a vague beauty benefit. It has actually cured a serious condition, and probably saved my life. In fact, I was told by a nutritionist recently that but for the brushing I would have eventually died in my own poison.'

Of course, regular skin brushing will not cure every serious liver complaint, and it should not be used as a substitute for medical care. But this story confirms what the skin-brushing enthusiasts claim – that the technique is far more than simply a beauty treatment, or something which makes you vaguely 'feel good'.

Daily skin brushing can help to stimulate far-reaching changes for the better within the body.

For cellulite removal though, it must be carried out in conjunction with the cleansing diet detailed in the previous chapter. There is no point in working hard to unclog the system from the outside if you are filling it up with rubbish on the inside.

Once the worst of the cellulite has gone, keep it away by occasional skin brushing once or twice a week. You don't want it to start creeping back after all your hard work.

Chapter 6

Aromatherapy

Most people regard aromatherapy as nothing more than a pleasantly relaxing beauty treatment. In fact, essential oils, as they are known, have extremely potent healing powers if used in the right way, and can encourage toxic wastes to disperse and be excreted. Far from being a mildly enjoyable indulgence, aromatherapy oils can enable an ill body or a sluggish system to return to a balanced and harmonious state.

Aromatherapy is the only branch of alternative medicine which really understands cellulite and treats it properly. Once we appreciate that the presence of cellulite is a visible indication of imbalance rather than actual fat, then we can begin to appreciate why and how aromatherapy works.

In her book *Aromatherapy: An A-Z* Patricia Davis says that 'aromatherapy is one of the most spectacularly successful forms of treatment for cellulite'.

The reason, I think, why so many people have been extremely cynical about the power of essential oils to reduce cellulite is because this condition is often attributed to overweight. Over the years there have been many claims that this or that cream, lotion or bodywrap could magically melt away fat. And in every single case where any such product has been subjected to independent investigation, its claims have not stood up at all.

Also aromatherapy has in recent years been very much confined to beauty treatments and beauty salons rather than hospitals or doctors' surgeries, which is why we have tended not to take it seriously. In fact, the science of treating illnesses with essential oils goes back thousands of years. The Ancient Greeks and Egyptians knew that many oils distilled from plants possessed potent therapeutic qualities, but the modern science of aromatherapy can be traced to the First World War, when Dr Jean Valnet, a French army surgeon, used essential oils to treat battle injuries and severe burns. He began to realize that the oils could be used to treat many kinds of illnesses, and after the war he used them on psychiatric patients. His book, *The Practice of Aromatherapy*, has become the standard textbook on the subject, and gives very specific details of how certain oils can help to reverse a wide variety of health problems. In everyday medicine, we use essential oils most often in the form of wintergreen ointment for aches and pains and oil of cloves for toothache.

It should be remembered that, until the advent of laboratory-produced chemical medicine this century, just about all remedies were based on plant materials, many of which have extremely powerful properties. Digitalis, derived from foxglove; heroin and morphine, from the opium poppy; and aspirin, from the willow tree, are all examples of strong medicines which come from plants. In modern times, evening primrose oil, aloe vera and ginseng have been advocated for a variety of health problems. And of course, very many plants can kill. Belladonna, from the deadly nightshade, hemlock and aconite are all examples of plants which can be fatal if you ingest them.

So we should not assume that an innocent-looking, exotic-smelling oil in a plain brown bottle has no healing power. In fact, now that people are becoming increasingly disillusioned with many laboratory-produced drugs because of their adverse side effects, there is an enormous upsurge of interest in natural remedies. This is probably the main reason why aromatherapy is now the fastest-growing of all branches of alternative medicine.

The word 'aromatherapy', like the word cellulite, is basically French, which may be why we in English-speaking countries have been slow to recognize it as a genuine branch of medicine. Aromatherapy can be used either as a beauty treatment, or to treat chronic and serious illness. Nowadays, a number of medical doctors in France are using scientific aromatherapy to treat sinus trouble, tonsillitis and catarrh, as well as for wound healing. Recent research at the Pasteur Institute has shown that certain oils can destroy mucus in the throat and elsewhere, and that aromatic oils can also considerably speed up wound healing. In France, a growing number of doctors are now using essential oils in place of laboratory-produced antibiotics, prescribing them as internal medicine, but you have to be medically qualified to prescribe them to be taken internally. Aromatherapists, as distinct from doctors, only ever use the oils for external purposes.

In France, there is now very well-documented evidence that several oils have powerful detoxifying qualities. It is now becoming increasingly accepted that illnesses result when poisons enter the system, in one form or another. When the body does not contain any poisonous material of any kind, whether this is manufactured inside the body, or comes in from outside, it will remain in perfect health.

It is true that aromatherapy treatments will not bring about any kind of weight loss, nor in themselves will they enable actual fat to shift. What they can do, however, is to encourage the accumulated toxic waste contained in fatty cells to disperse and be eliminated through the kidneys, liver and skin. They do this because certain essential oils have the power to stimulate body systems which may have become sluggish and less than maximally efficient.

WHAT ARE ESSENTIAL OILS?

Basically they are the strong-smelling ingredients found in many plants. They provide the distinctive aroma you get when you bruise a lavender, sage or rosemary leaf, for instance. Most flowers, seeds, grains, roots and resins contain essential oils in minute quantities.

Some of these oils are healing, and some are harmful. Harmful essential oils include wormwood, as used in absinthe. Healing oils include rosemary, geranium, patchouli, lavender, and sweet almond. Oils from plants become 'essential' after they have been distilled, and the highly concentrated 'essence' is obtained. As very little oil is obtained from each plant, the concentrated form of essential oils is very expensive indeed.

Once the oils have been distilled they are very volatile and will quickly evaporate. This is why you always find aromatherapy oils in dark blue or brown bottles to keep the destructive effect of light away from their contents.

Chemically speaking, these oils are very complicated, and this is where their therapeutic power lies. They are readily absorbed through the skin, and taken up into the bloodstream. Sometimes they can have a very quick effect indeed. I have spoken to some cellulite sufferers who have had to get up off the couch and go to the toilet whilst having the oils rubbed in by an aromatherapist.

Certain oils have a diuretic effect, some are relaxing, while others are stimulating and energizing. Just to give a few examples – clary sage is a powerful relaxant and helps digestion; geranium is an adrenal cortex stimulant and reliever of fluid retention; lavender is calming and soothing; cypress is a powerful astringent; juniper purifies and stimulates the urino-genital tract. Rosemary encourages the lymphatic system to start working properly.

There are literally hundreds of essential oils and it would take years to learn how to use them all properly. But you do not need to be a qualified aromatherapist mixing up mysterious oils to enable them to release their powerful alchemy. Luckily, much of the work has already been done for the cellulite sufferer, so all you have to do is make sure you buy the right kind of oils and use them correctly.

There are two ways of using aromatherapy to combat cellulite. You can either do it yourself, or you can go to a qualified therapist. Some will find it nicer and perhaps more self-disciplinary to go to a therapist, but it is perfectly possible to use the oils all by yourself to help the cellulite to disappear.

SELF HELP

There are now a number of special anti-cellulite oils on the market which are based on aromatherapy principles. These are not the highly expensive 'miracle creams' but a mixture of essential oils diluted in the correct carrier oils. You can either buy anti-cellulite oils ready mixed, or make up your own from small bottles of essential oils.

The two main manufacturers of organic anti-cellulite oils in the UK are **Bodytreats International** and **Neal's Yard**.

Bodytreats have two types of anti-cellulite oils: a bath oil and a massage oil. The bath oil contains 'neat' essential oil for the bath, and the massage oil is a dilution of the same oils in a vegetable carrier oil. You should put one to five drops (never more) into the bath.

Neal's Yard have a differently formulated anti-cellulite oil, containing lemon, frankincense, juniper, black pepper and sandalwood in a base oil. Their leaflet states that the oil will help to 'eliminate toxins developing in the fatty tissues and in the body'. Black pepper is a very hot essential oil and you may find yourself tingling after massaging in this particular anti-cellulite treatment.

Please see the Appendix for details on how to mix your own anti-cellulite oils.

You can dissolve any greasiness left by the oils on clothing by prewashing in liquid soda, available in supermarkets.

USE OF THE OILS

After body brushing in the way described in the previous chapter, shake between one and five drops of essential oil (*not* the massage oil) into the bath. Lie there, if possible, for about a quarter of an hour, breathing deeply and letting the concentrated oil do its work. As you lie in the bath, knead and pummel the cellulite-heavy areas. You will soon get to know which these are.

Then, after getting out of the bath and drying yourself, massage a small amount of the diluted oil into each thigh, and the buttocks. You can do this with your hands, paying particular attention to the cellulite areas, or with a loofah. Also rub a tiny amount of the oil over your stomach to increase detoxification, and then get dressed. The oils will take about ten minutes to be absorbed completely, and there will be no residual 'oiliness' on your skin after this time. The oils should not spoil or stain clothes if you rub them in sufficiently.

It is best to perform the anti-cellulite treatments either first thing in the morning or, if you don't have time then, in the early evening. Don't do it last thing at night, not because there is anything inherently dangerous in the programme but because the combination of skin brushing, bath and massage will probably keep you awake, as the overall effect is extremely stimulating.

At first you should do the body brushing, aromatherapy and massage every day. Then, after about three or four weeks, use the massage oils every other day. When most of the cellulite has dispersed – and you will know this by your new sleek outline and lack of dimples – use the body brush plus the oils just once or twice a week.

As you progress with the treatment you will probably notice that previously hard areas of thigh and buttock have become soft and flabby. Now, you may think that flab is as bad as cellulite, but actually it's not. This kind of flab is a temporary condition brought about when the fatty cells are emptied of their excess water content. Brisk massage and exercise plus continued use of the aromatherapy oils will tone up the flab, and you will soon notice it firming up.

Do keep the measure handy to measure your thighs. There will soon be a visible difference, if you apply the oils conscientiously and regularly. Some people don't like measuring themselves. I'm one of them. In this case, keep a skinny pair of trousers or pencil skirt to get into when your cellulite disappears, and you will soon see the difference.

Don't be surprised if your shape starts to change. You may discover than your waist or ankles change. The backs of the calves can be quite resistant to treatment, and may need extra-vigorous massage.

And do allow yourself time – don't expect everything to happen all at once. Frances Clifford has said:

'People come crying to me in desperation, and have been led to believe the cellulite will disappear overnight. It won't – especially for those women who, like most of my clients, have been bothered by cellulite for many years.'

If you do decide to treat your cellulite yourself, make sure you use only the proper aromatherapy oils, or anti-cellulite oils blended on aromatherapy principles. Don't be tempted to spend large sums of money on creams which are supposed to 'improve circulation'. They will not help a cellulite problem to any great extent.

In her article on cellulite in *The Sunday Times* Maggie Drummond wondered what might happen to the fat if these creams worked. Was it shifted elsewhere, she asked, or might it disappear altogether? In any case, she could not understand how the creams could possibly make an iota of difference. 'Do I believe that a contour cream is what it takes for a slimmer, trimmer thigh?' she wrote. 'Pull the other one. It's got gingko biloba tree extract on it.'

In other words, scepticism was absolute. Until it is generally known and accepted that cellulite is a quite different problem from ordinary excess fat, this kind of unhelpful confusion will continue.

Note: although aromatherapy oils are extremely effective at getting rid of cellulite, *they will not work unless you also stick to the diet*. There is not much point in going to all the trouble and expense of aromatherapy treatments if you continue to smoke, drink and eat junk, for as fast as you are getting rid of accumulated toxic wastes, new ones are entering the body.

GOING TO A THERAPIST

Women who have huge amounts of cellulite, or fear that they may lack the willpower and motivation to give themselves regular treatments, may be better off going to a qualified therapist who has had proven success in treating cellulite.

When booking up an aromatherapist, ask her to give you the names of people who have already been treated, and speak to them. No reputable therapist will mind putting you in touch with grateful clients – in fact, very many aromatherapists never advertise, but get new customers simply by word of mouth.

When speaking to women who have been successfully treated, ask how long it took, what it cost, and how the treatment progressed. Then, if you feel satisfied, book up six sessions. For most people, this should be enough to get rid of the worst of the problem. However, in my own case, six sessions of extremely hard massage with the oils hardly made any difference and I had to book up more treatments. You will usually be advised to have two treatments a week – they are more effective when coming close together.

Usually the first treatment will consist of a consultation, where the therapist will ask important questions about general health, varicose veins, any pills or medical treatment you may be having. If you have high blood pressure, or any other serious or chronic illness such as a heart condition, asthma, or a recurring skin condition, you should see a therapist rather than attempt to treat the cellulite by yourself. Certain oils are contra-indicated if there are chronic health problems.

The therapist will explain that, however hard she works to pummel away the cellulite deposits, at least sixty per cent of the work must come from you, the patient. You have to make up your mind to stick to the diet, which may consist of nothing but mineral water and fresh fruits for about three days, to begin the detoxifying process. After that, you can gradually add more foods, making sure always that your diet consists mainly of natural wholefoods. You will be much better off if you can manage a completely vegetarian diet, as this is far less toxic than a meat one.

For the actual therapy sessions the practitioner will ask you to take off all your clothes except pants and bra – and will then inspect and assess the cellulite. A vigorous massage session will follow, lasting for about half an hour. If the cellulite is really bad or deep, this massage may hurt. A therapist who has been trained in lymphatic drainage massage will really dig in. You will know when she reaches the cellulite points as there may be a moment of sharp pain. During the initial sessions, you may find your legs are covered in bruises afterwards.

Remember that drastic changes will be taking place inside your body as the cellulite disperses, and these may be accompanied by insomnia, outbreaks of spots and a slight fluctuation in menstrual patterns, mood changes and negative feelings. You may get colds and flu, catarrh, and headaches. Tissues may be very tender at first. You may also get headaches, perhaps as bad as migraine. But don't worry. These are all signs of toxic matter clearing itself out of your system.

The worse the cellulite, the more dramatic the changes will be, but all the nasty side effects will disappear before long. As the treatments proceed, you will feel and become quite a different person. Your body image and self-esteem will be raised, and you will certainly notice higher energy levels, as the toxins are released from the system.

My therapist, Frances Clifford, used a mixture of cypress, lavender, juniper berry and clary sage on my cellulite and found that after eight treatments it started moving really quickly. When I first went along, my legs were a solid mass of cellulite, but eventually this was reduced to isolated pockets here and there. These 'pockets' were extremely resistant, as they had probably been there for a very long time, but eventually they too started to disperse.

Removing cellulite can be likened to getting rid of rust, or cleaning up silver that has been neglected for a long time. The longer it has been left, the more difficult the job, but in every case, if you persevere for long enough, the tarnish and rust will go. You just need enough elbow grease and the right rust-dissolving preparation.

As the treatment proceeds, most therapists will keep quite detailed case notes, to enable them to keep a check on progress. A reputable therapist will be able to tell you whether you have a water retention problem in addition to the cellulite. Usually, though, you will know this because water retention means thick, spongy ankles. There are, of course, aromatherapy treatments which can combat this problem but they are slightly different. For one thing, the type of massage used will be far lighter and gentler.

All aromatherapists have different ways of treating cellulite, though the overall understanding of the condition is the same. Patricia Davis uses a combination of detoxifying and lymphatic-system-stimulating oils, plus those which have mildly diuretic properties. She says that as the treatment will possibly need to be continued over several weeks or even months, depending on the extent of the cellulite, it is important to vary the oils. As with any medicines, the body gets used to the same oils after a time, and they lose their effectiveness.

Patricia usually begins treatment with a combination of geranium and rosemary in equal proportions, and incorporates a small amount of black pepper, juniper and fennel.

Another aromatherapist, Danièle Ryman, uses a mixture of cypress, lavender and lemon, and advises drinking sage and vervain teas.

Also, as people are themselves very individual, they may react differently to the oils. I found that the Bodytreats anti-cellulite oils were extremely stimulating, and kept me awake if I used them too late at night. A good therapist will discover the range of oils which are just right for your particular condition, general health status, age, skin type and temperament.

Whether you decide to enlist the help of a therapist or go it alone it is important to regard cellulite removal as a medical treatment, in much the same way as you would approach getting rid of acne, eczema, migraine, or any other chronic condition which makes you feel miserable and depressed.

All aromatherapists recognize that there is a significant stress component in cellulite, and that the condition is far more likely to form at times of tension and anxiety. This is why it is very common for cellulite to be laid down when young women first leave home to go to university or college, embark on a disastrous love affair, have to tackle difficult exams or projects at work, or give up a career to bring up children. Any prolonged stressful event can encourage cellulite to form, as all poisons are more readily held in the system when there is a state of stress.

A good aromatherapist will recognize this, and combine the vigorous massage with a calm-down massage before the treatment finishes. The total effect of the treatments is to leave you in a calmer and more confident state.

Perhaps these sound like large claims to make for a treatment which appears to consist simply of having a variety of fragrant and exotic oils rubbed into your legs. But to my mind the proof of the pudding is in the eating. Many, many women in this country have removed their cellulite by this means, and are successfully keeping it off.

PREPARING YOUR OWN ANTI-CELLULITE OILS

You should always match up bath oils to massage oils when embarking on anti-cellulite treatments. Essential oils which are good to put in the bath include lemon, rosemary, geranium, patchouli, cypress or juniper. These are all equally effective, and can be bought as single oils from any supplier of aromatherapy products such as Neal's Yard, Culpeper, or Bodytreats.

Lemon has an alkalizing effect on body systems, cypress is good for those who have any problems with their veins, and juniper is particularly effective for people who smoke or who have to travel or work in crowded, smoky environments.

You should shake six to ten drops of the essential oil into the bath and relax in the water for about fifteen minutes. After you have dried yourself, massage in the massage oils. These can easily be made by filling a 100 ml bottle – it should be opaque and dark – with the base or carrier oil, and then shaking about thirty drops of the essential oil into this.

The base, or carrier, oil that you use is important. It should be pure vegetable oil such as sweet almond, apricot kernel, avocado (very rich), grapeseed, hazelnut or sunflower. Ordinary kitchen cooking oil will do so long as it is not blended, and is cold-pressed. If it is cold-pressed, it will say so on the label. You can use olive oil if you like, although this is rather strong-smelling. But it works perfectly well as a carrier oil.

Remember that the massage action is as important as the oil itself, so rub it in as hard as you can.

Some essential oils are not suitable for anti-cellulite treatments. These include all the spice oils and most of the flower oils, which have no effect whatever. The best ones to use are the herb oils or the tree oils, as these work to improve circulation and are also invigorating and toning. Each essential oil, like each herb, has a specific quality and not all are equally good.

You can also burn oils to inhale the fragrance. Oil burners can be bought from most craftshops and fill the air with a wonderful fragrance which has potent de-stressing qualities. Lavender, which helps to take acid out of the system, is good for burning whenever you feel tense and anxious, but any of the oils listed above will do the same job. Six drops are all you need to release the fragrance. This can be done whenever you don't have time for a bath, and should be done as often as you can, as one of the causes of cellulite is, of course, undue stress.

Do remember whenever embarking on anti-cellulite treatments never to sit with crossed legs. This cuts off circulation and encourages cellulite to form. Try to get into the habit of sitting with legs straight, and with ankles higher than hips whenever possible.

IMPORTANT: You should never use the same oils for more than two or three weeks at a time, as they lose their potency once the body gets used to them. In this, they are exactly like any other drug. For rapid effect, change your oils frequently. For instance, if you use cypress for the first three weeks, change to rosemary for the next three weeks. The body likes to be surprised and stimulated.

BOTANICAL NAMES OF ANTI-CELLULITE AROMATHERAPY OILS

- LEMON: *Citrus limonum*
- JUNIPER: *Juniperus communis* ssp. *communis*
- ROSEMARY: *Rosmarinus officinalis* CT cineole
- CLARY SAGE: *Salvia sclarea*
- CYPRESS: *Cupressus sempervirens*
- PATCHOULI: *Pogostemon cablin*
- GERANIUM: *Pelargonium* x *asperum (roseum)*

Two other essential oils may be used for anti-cellulite. These are BLACK PEPPER (*Piper nigrum*; this oil is good for people who are particularly sensitive to cold, and in winter) and SANDALWOOD (*Santalum album*; this acts as a lymphatic decongestant, and is relaxing as well).

Chapter 7

The Benefits of Massage

Massage is the final important ingredient of any successful cellulite-removing regime. If you are carrying out a self-help programme you should always make sure you massage the oils in well after a bath, rather than just rubbing them in.

First of all, pour a little massage oil – about a teaspoonful – into the palm of your hand, and rub it slightly into your hands. You should never pour any oils directly onto the skin. Then with long stroking movements start at the ankle and work up to the knee and thigh. Use both hands and make sure the movements are gentle but firm. This type of massage encourages circulation and can stimulate blood flow.

A good type of massage for cellulite-laden areas is **kneading**, which is also known by masseurs as *pétrissage*. For this, you have to pretend you are kneading a loaf of bread as you pick up the flesh and squeeze it, applying as much pressure as you can. It is rather like pinching huge areas of flesh.

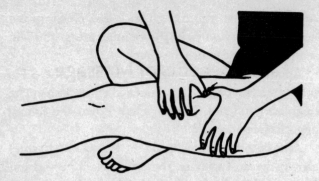

kneading

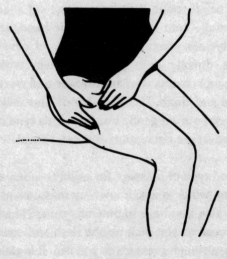

rolling

After doing this, you can go back and pinch up the flesh in the very worst of the cellulite areas. You will soon get to know which these are.

Another useful movement for cellulite sufferers is **rolling**. Here, you pick up about an inch of flesh on the thigh and roll the flesh to break down the lumpy deposits (see diagram).

After a time you will get to know which areas contain the most cellulite. They will feel ridgy, hard and grainy, and you will experience a ripply sensation as you learn to apply more pressure. Long-ingrained cellulite will feel like rows of chipolatas when you massage. These are the areas to concentrate on, as the cellulite will need a lot of encouragement to go. Whenever you are massaging your thigh and come across an area which feels particularly tender you can be sure this is where the cellulite is at its worst.

Once you feel you have got to know your cellulite, you can dig at it with your thumb, using as much pressure as you are able to. Now you have embarked on an anti-cellulite programme, any kind of kneading and pinching and pounding will only do good.

Make sure you knead and pound the lumpy areas when you are lying in the bath, especially if you have shaken in a few drops of concentrated essential oils. You can also knead and wring the spare flesh at any time of day – whenever you have a few moments of privacy. From now on any kind of attention, such as stroking, rolling, kneading or wringing, will have good effects and you will soon start seeing the difference.

Daily massaging helps you to get to know the cellulite areas, and you will also become acquainted with your whole body in a way you never did before. But when you pummel away at the lumpy areas, don't do it with hatred. Very many women – myself included for a long time – feel only disgust when they look down at their thighs, and start hating their legs. When massaging, you should treat the thighs with loving care, reminding yourself that you are doing your very best for them, to enable them to lose the rubbish the fat cells have held for so long. In the same way that some people speak to plants, therapists often advise their clients to start talking to their cellulite, and to try and visualize it seeping out of fatty cells as they knead and pound away at the bulgy areas. It may sound ridiculous at first, but visualization has become a very popular therapy for cancer patients in America. Some clinics advise patients to use their imagination and see the tumours shrinking as they concentrate on their cancer.

Now, I'm not for one minute suggesting that cellulite is a problem on the same level as cancer, but it is unwanted and unhealthy just the same. Visualization can be very effective when you are massaging, as it helps you to concentrate hard on the cellulite areas, rather than going off into a day dream.

Whenever you are alone, watching television, or otherwise relaxing, put your legs in the air one at a time, and gently stroke up them, starting at the ankle and going right up to the hip joint. This encourages the lymphatic system to become more active, and also helps toxic wastes to start draining away.

It is the regularity of the massage which makes the difference. At first, when the cellulite is very bad, you should make sure you do it every single day. The order is: body brushing, bath (with drops of essential oils), then massaging in the oils. At first, it may seem extremely self-indulgent to spend so much time on yourself every day, but the rewards will soon be noticed in disappearing cellulite.

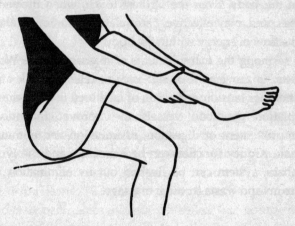

During the past few years, there has been an enormous upsurge of interest in massage techniques. It is now at last being accepted that all types of massage, from gentle stroking to hard pounding and pummelling, can have enormous beneficial effects on the whole system. Like aromatherapy, massage used to be regarded rather as a self-indulgent beauty treatment, something which was medically neither here nor there.

Now we know differently. Pioneering masseuses such as Clare Maxwell-Hudson have shown that the ancient art of massage can be at least as effective as much modern medicine, and can bring about dramatic changes in the body. American masseuse Ouida West says in her book, *The Magic of Massage*, 'I define massage as any touch that is capable of evoking a change in the body. Even the lightest touch, when properly executed, may effectively stimulate circulation or alter the flow of energy within the body.'

Among the many benefits of massage Ouida West lists: improvement of self-esteem; relief of neck and shoulder tension; reduction of fat stored in the tissues; dilation of blood vessels to improve circulation; improvement of digestion, assimilation and elimination. Kidney function can be increased, and the lymphatic system can be flushed out by elimination of toxins and waste through massage.

TAKE TIME FOR YOURSELF

Women who live by themselves are lucky when embarking on an anti-cellulite regime, because they can please themselves what they eat, when they massage, and when they have their bath. Those who are married, have a family, or share a flat may not be so fortunate, because it has to be admitted that those you live with will, on the whole, resent the time you take for yourself. You may also have to cope with comments such as: 'but you're quite thin enough as you are', or 'but I like your legs like that.' This type of remark is most often passed by the man in one's life. Men can particularly get annoyed when the women in their life go off and massage and pummel their thighs.

The strength of mind needed to combat cellulite successfully should never be over-estimated. You just have to make up your mind not to hear these remarks, and carry on, even while others may tell you – usually without knowing the first thing about the subject themselves – that it's a complete waste of time and money. I know from experience that you have to be completely single-minded when deciding to banish cellulite. Like an unwelcome guest, it never wants to go, and will take up permanent squatter's rights in your body whenever it can. You just have to regard it in the same way as household dust and dirt – something you must continually struggle to keep down.

Daily massage is really essential, so do make sure you make time to include it in your general routine. Occasional pummellings and kneadings are not enough.

Although very many massage books on the market speak enthusiastically about people learning to do massage for each other, I have very strong doubts about whether this really works. Mostly, people are encouraged to massage each other for sexual or intimate reasons, and with cellulite-removal this is the last thing on your mind. You are carrying out a self-help medical treatment, not indulging in sexual foreplay. For this reason, I would say that it is not a good idea for a husband, boyfriend or lover to try and help you get rid of your cellulite. For one thing, most of them couldn't care a hoot whether you have cellulite or not, and for another, the intimate kind of stroking needed could soon take a sexual turn. Having said this, it can be difficult to apply the kind of pressure needed on the backs of your thighs by yourself. So, if you can persuade somebody to do it for you – with firmness and kindness, so as not to hurt – then this will speed up results.

If you have friends who are professional masseurs, or who have taken courses, then that is a different thing. But I can't think it would be a good idea to entrust your body to somebody who doesn't know what they are doing. It's far better to do it by yourself, and take responsibility for yourself.

GOING TO A THERAPIST

If you are considering going to a professional, make sure you choose somebody who is qualified to practise both aromatherapy and lymphatic drainage. It is important to ask about the lymphatic draining, because this will be your clue that the therapist really can help you. If you get a confused silence on the end of the phone when you ask your local aromatherapist about this kind of massage, then don't book her up. Also ask, of course, about the nutritional aspects, as no massage alone, however tough, can disperse cellulite. It is essential that your therapist should understand exactly what cellulite is.

LYMPHATIC DRAINAGE MASSAGE

This is a highly specialized technique whereby the masseuse activates the main lymph nodes in order to get them working again. She does this by pressing on the lymph points all over your body and applying pressure to them. Although you would probably need to go to a professional to get a proper lymphatic drainage, you can easily learn for yourself where the main lymph nodes are, and press these after you have finished the kneading and pounding massage.

The diagram overleaf shows where the main points are – under the armpits, in the thoracic duct between the breasts, in the lumbar region, behind the knees. It won't take long to learn where these are, and touching them will definitely help the lymphatic system to get working properly again.

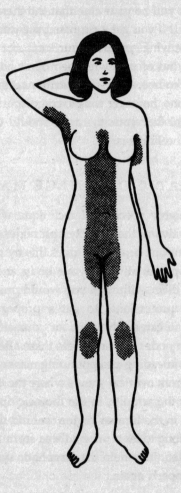

Some people find that when the body is really over-loaded with toxic and waste matter the lymph nodes feel tender. If this is the case with you, don't give up, but keep applying gentle pressure until the tenderness ceases. As you carry on with the regime, you will find that the nodes become less tender. Tenderness in these regions means that there is a blockage, and it may take time for this to be released.

Those who are going to a therapist should always say when they feel any pain or tenderness in any area whatever. You can't expect her to be a mind reader, although an experienced therapist will be aware of possible tender points.

A professional anti-cellulite massage will usually take between half and three-quarters of an hour, and the therapist will concentrate only on the cellulite areas and the lymphatic points. She will not usually give you a general massage, and she will not touch your back or your front. You can of course, if you like, ask for a general massage, but this is a different kind of treatment.

The advantage of going to a therapist is that an objective check will be kept on your progress, but don't imagine that all is lost if you cannot find anybody suitable in your area. At the time of writing, there are not many people trained in this form of massage who have also studied the vital nutritional and dietary aspects, which is one of the reasons I'm writing this book! Once you have the information at your finger-tips, and can understand exactly what cellulite is and

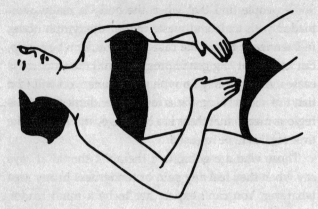

what is needed to remove it, you can effectively become your own therapist.

Most professionals finish up by stroking the abdomen gently in circular movements. This aids the digestive system, and also helps waste products to disperse. It is easy enough to do this for yourself, using a tiny trace of oil. Make sure the movements are extremely gentle here.

When a professional massage has been completed, you will usually be asked to lie still on the couch for a few minutes to collect yourself. Lymphatic drainage massage can be very hard and tough, and you may feel slightly faint if you get up instantly. If you are doing your own massage, take a tip from the professionals, and lie down for a little while after you have finished. I can guarantee that you will feel quite wonderful when you get up.

The timing of daily self-massage is important. You probably won't have time to do it properly first thing in the morning, and last thing at night the whole exercise can be far too stimulating. So the optimum time is early evening, before supper. If you can get into the habit of performing the anti-cellulite massage at this time you will definitely have renewed energy for the evening, and will not be tempted to fill yourself up with snacks and junk foods.

One of the benefits of massage is that, after you have been cosseting and caring for your body on the outside in this way, you feel much less like putting rubbish into the inside. By massaging yourself, you learn to respect your body, both inside and out.

You will also notice other benefits from regular massage with essential oils. Your skin and clothes will become delicately impregnated with the fragrance of the oils, and also your skin will become softer and smoother. You are likely to have fewer headaches, to feel less irritable and touchy, and less stressed generally.

Anything which reduces stress is to be recommended because, of course, there is a major stress element in the development of cellulite. The less tense and anxious you are, the less cellulite will be formed. This is not just some airy-fairy notion but a scientifically acknowledged fact. When the mind is tense and anxious extra stress hormones (adrenalin) are released into the system, and stay there. The more chronic the stress, the greater the release of adrenalin and the greater, eventually, the build-up of toxic wastes.

Digestion, elimination and circulation are all adversely affected by mental stress. We are only just learning – or appreciating – how closely linked the mind and body are, and how intimately the feedback principle operates. Whatever affects the mind will soon reverberate in the body, and vice versa. Massage is a potent means of unstressing the system, and thus counteracting the production of excess adrenalin.

As we know, the formation of cellulite is basically an elimination problem, so anything which helps body systems to return to normal will also aid reduction of these wastes.

WHAT ABOUT EXERCISE?

As most cellulite sufferers know only too well, no amount of exercise will shift even a millimetre of cellulite. This doesn't mean you shouldn't be physically active, of course, only that you should not even begin to rely on exercise to get rid of the lumps and bumps.

We know, of course, that the formation of cellulite is associated with leading a sedentary life, which in turn means that circulation is likely to be poor. So exercise can very much help to *prevent* cellulite. If you look at leading female athletes you will notice that not one of them has even the tiniest trace of cellulite. All have legs which look as if they are made from the lightest and best-tempered steel, with not an ounce of flab or spare flesh. Because these women have been athletes ever since they were children, it is unlikely that cellulite ever had a chance to lay itself down.

The time to embark on exercise is once the cellulite has started to disappear. As soon as you begin an anti-cellulite programme, you should make up your mind to become as physically active as possible. This means walking instead of taking a bus or the lift at work and going for a swim whenever possible. Any gentle, rhythmic form of exercise will help to keep circulation moving, which is what you are aiming at.

Once you are left with residual flab, after the worst of the cellulite has made its exit, you can do the tried and tested bicycling in the air, copy somebody who does routines on breakfast television, or book keep-fit classes at a local gym. Local-authority-run keep-fit and conditioning classes are extremely cheap, and usually very good.

Yoga exercises will also firm up flabby muscles, if you are that way inclined. Although yoga classes will help to put a long-misused body back into alignment, the movements are too slow and sustained to be of enormous help in muscle toning. Yoga positions will certainly help you to find out where the cellulite-laden areas are, and enable you to realize where stiffness and lack of suppleness lie, but they are not specifically designed to firm up the flab left when cellulite makes its exit.

The good thing about yoga positions, or *asanas* as they are known, is that by doing them – or at least attempting them – you get to know and respect your own body. The other valuable aspect of yoga is that it is not harmful in any way, as perhaps aerobics or California-stretch-type classes might be.

What you should never do is attempt a vigorous work-out if you have been completely sedentary for years on end. This is as much a shock to the system as a drastically altered diet and the body may not be able to cope. Many women find that, once they have got rid of the worst of the cellulite, they have a far more positive attitude to their bodies and no longer fear putting on a leotard or joining an exercise class. This is good – but don't be tempted to overdo it at first. Apart from anything else, you'll never keep it up. It is far better to start with a very gentle exercise regime intended for beginners, and then gradually become more vigorous as your body can take it.

There are now many multi-gyms around the country, and also all kinds of exercise machines you can buy for yourself.

The great majority of people use exercise bikes and the like for a short time and then become bored and forget about them. If you suspect this is you, don't be tempted to spend vast sums of money on expensive home gyms. It would be far better for you to attend weekly sessions at a commercial gym, where your progress will be monitored.

Of course, after you have completed an anti-cellulite programme, your body and general health will be far better than before, and you will probably feel much more like doing exercise. To be effective, any exercise has to be regular, and you will never keep it up unless you enjoy it. You should walk or swim at least three times a week and, ideally, go to keep-fit classes twice a week. Exercise experts have worked out that, in order to do any good, your chosen form of exercise should be practised at least three times a week, and for at least twenty minutes at a time. Any less, and you might as well not bother.

However, if you get rid of the cellulite first, by being conscientious about the regime outlined in this book, and then complete the good work by the right kind of exercise, you will – I promise you – be rewarded by the kind of figure and good health you had never previously dreamed possible.

It happened to me. And if I, as a lifelong exercise-hater and self-indulgent soul, can get rid of cellulite after more than twenty years, so can you.

Personal note: After I finished my anti-cellulite treatments, I first of all had a personal trainer, which worked wonders to firm up the flabby muscles, but after a time that became too expensive. It's also rather lonely. Then I tried yoga for a time, but eventually found this both too boring and too difficult. For several years now I have gone to a strenuous exercise class two or three times a week.

I vary this, doing sometimes step, sometimes tums, bums and thighs, sometimes high- and low-impact aerobics. The result of this is that my leg muscles have acquired definition and, although not quite in the elite athlete class, look strong and sinewy rather than flabby and jelly-like.

There's no doubt that a defined body looks better in clothes (as well as out of them!) and if you can possibly keep up an exercise regime like this, you won't be disappointed. The other bonus, of course, is that you'll feel so much better than if you don't exercise.

Chapter 8

New Research, Evidence and Products

When this book first appeared, most doctors in Britain and America were extremely scornful of the whole idea of cellulite, which, they firmly believed, was simply another way that get-rich-quick cosmetic companies were conning vain, credulous women. There was no real evidence, they maintained, to suggest that cellulite existed as a separate entity to or was in any way different from ordinary fat.

Now, though, the tide is turning. Although it would not be true to say that every single doctor accepts the existence of these toxic wastes, at least *some* medically-qualified people (and not just in France) now believe that the evidence for its reality has become overwhelming.

Two British consultant dermatologists who have become convinced about cellulite are Dr Roger Dawbey and Dr Terence Ryan, both of the Department of Dermatology, Slade Hospital, Headington in Oxford.

Dr Ryan, co-editor of the textbook *Cutaneous Adipose Tissue*, believes that cellulite can no longer be considered

an invention of French cosmetic companies. He says
that this form of fluid retention has been almost
completely neglected by the medical profession until
recently, partly because it was not a painful condition
(and therefore not something that people would readily take to the doctor), and partly because there have
been no medical cures or effective treatments available. For these reasons there has been very little proper
academic research into the subject.

Dr Ryan also points out that dermatologists have in
the past given little serious attention to cellulite
because they have not wanted to seem too gullible or
too readily taken in by the claims and hype of the
cosmetic industry. Nor, he says, have serious doctors
wanted to align themselves with purely cosmetic doctors, as this may well have meant they would not be
taken seriously by other members of their profession.

In his chapter 'Panniculopathy and Fibrosclerosis of
the Female Breast and Thigh', Dr Ryan defines cellulite
as basically a disorder of adipose – fat – tissue. What
has happened, he says, is that there is 'segmented and
localized lipodystrophy of the subcutaneous connective tissue', which in layperson's terms means that a
degeneration of fat cells has occurred, causing the
lumps and bumps we know as cellulite. Dr Ryan
admits that 'cellulite' is an unsatisfactory term, as this
is not an inflammatory disorder and because the term
has been adopted and popularized by the cosmetic
industry, which does not endear it to the medical

profession. But, like others, he accepts that the term will probably have to remain in use, simply because there is no other.

Studies by leading dermatologists in America have, he says, identified cellulite as being caused by a malfunction of the lymphatic system – which is what aromatherapists and other complementary practitioners were saying years ago, only to be shouted down by orthodoxy for propounding such cranky nonsense.

The lumps and bumps start to appear, says Dr Ryan, because fluid which should be draining away is instead collecting around the capillaries supplying individual fat cells. In one research project, a total of 48 biopsies taken from women complaining of cellulite showed that their skin and underlying adipose tissue had hardened and degenerated owing to lengthy accumulation of this fluid. As women got older, the problem seemed to become worse, as ever more fluid accumulated, and it became increasingly more difficult for it to drain away.

Cellulite is not exactly a problem of ageing – it's just that as we get older the problem keeps getting worse. Gradual sclerosis leads to micronodule formation – which is a medical man's way of describing the 'orange peel' appearance known and hated by all cellulite sufferers.

The 'cold' feel of cellulite, Dr Ryan says, is caused by fluid accumulation leading to a gradual impairment of blood flow to the area.

Dr Ryan also believes that high intakes of saturated fat are implicated in the formation of cellulite. And certainly it is observable that cellulite is always worst in countries where saturated fats form a significant part of the diet. France, which has pioneered research into cellulite, has a national diet extremely high in saturated fats and dairy products, while in Japan, where cellulite is hardly ever seen, most fats consumed are polyunsaturated. Saturated fats, it is believed, bind up water to give the appearance of oedema. The dermis – the deep layer of the skin – gradually loses elasticity, and the lymphatic drainage mechanism cannot operate efficiently. The result of this is a Sargasso sea of trapped fluid and toxic deposits, none of which will go away without determined help.

In common with other doctors who have taken the problem seriously, Dr Ryan believes that the best way of ridding these fluids from the system is regular massage. Cellulite, he believes, is a sign of premature ageing – something which has also been noted by a number of French researchers. Cellulite is, in fact, the visible warning sign that the cells in these areas are undergoing faster degeneration than those in other places. The lumps and bumps are actually a sign that cells are rapidly ageing under the onslaught of rapidly accumulating fluids.

The art historian Kenneth Clark said in his classic book, *The Nude*, that the reason cellulite offends (not that he gave it that name) is because it is not smooth.

When curvature gives way to lumps and bumps we find it ugly, he stated.

French doctors have, of course, been pre-eminent in the study of cellulite. Unfortunately, their work has not attained enormous credibility in other countries partly because we have been so very resistant to the idea of cellulite until recently, and partly because their work has almost always been funded by major cosmetic or pharmaceutical companies. For this reason, it has not been seen as independent research. Of course there are difficulties in accepting work carried out by scientists which has been financed by a profitmaking company anxious to market new products. But the fact is that most modern scientific research – into AIDS, cancer, arthritis or any other serious modern disease – is financed by drug companies, and cannot all be dismissed on that account.

The latest research instigated by Pierre Fabre, whose Elancyl products are the market leaders in anti-cellulite treatments, and have been for thirty years, supports that endorsed by Dr Terence Ryan. Doctors and scientists from the University of Toulouse have discovered, using highly sophisticated thermographic instruments, that cellulite is the gradual accumulation of fluid and toxic matter in the connective tissues.

When cellulite starts to accumulate, the connective tissues in the fat cells are irritated and begin to harden. The effect of this is to compress the blood vessels, cutting off circulation and preventing the normal biological processes, such as the operation of the lymphatic system, from doing their jobs of eliminating the unwanted materials. Instead of being carried away as they should be, the fluid and toxic matter continue to build up around the connective tissues. These migrate to the dermis, where they remain and harden. The result is the dreaded orange peel or mattress skin – something no woman should have to put up with.

If the mass is merely fat, as opposed to cellulite, say the researchers, the skin remains smooth. Fat by itself will never cause the lumpy, bumpy appearance characterizing cellulite. The difference between obesity and cellulite is that with the former the fatty cells can move freely; they are not blocked. With cellulite, by contrast, the fat cells are trapped in connective tissue, and this is why cellulite-laden areas feel hard and knobbly, not soft like ordinary fat areas.

Although cellulite is not exactly fat, it is caused by a serious malfunction of the fat cells. One possible reason women are more prone to this condition than men (apart from the hormonal aspect, which is accepted by most doctors working in this area) is that women have twice the amount of fatty tissue of men, and the ability of their fat cells to multiply is twice as great. There is also far more connective tissue in women's bodies, according to the latest research into adipose tissue.

This much is known about cellulite – it is no longer a matter for conjecture and theory. Detailed research in France has also established that a brown, rank, smelly, oily substance with no known physiological function has been found in cellulite-laden cells.

One French definition of cellulite is: 'Large, distorted, adipocyte agglomerations which merge together, changing from the adipocyte in its normal state to the random accumulation of peroxodase fats destroying the adipocytes'! In plain English, this means just what we have already said, that the accumulation of unwanted material in the fatty cells causes premature degeneration of the tissues.

In time, the fats oxidize, causing the smelly, oily substance. New research on cellulite has been made possible by ultrasonic tomography, a method of looking at a cross-section of the skin without damaging the tissues. The research has also established that cellulite, once it has made its appearance, will never disappear of its own accord.

Once it has been noticed, say the French researchers, it needs very specific treatment. Otherwise, the ever-increasing accumulation of toxins in these areas will cause premature ageing, loss of skin elasticity, fluid retention and oedema.

Scientific research has also now confirmed that cellulite arises very largely from oestrogen imbalance. There are particular danger times when female hormones are particularly active, such as at puberty (cellulite is rare, if not unknown, before adolescence), when the Pill is taken, during pregnancy and at the menopause. According to research commissioned by

Pierre Fabre, 75 per cent of cellulite is laid down when there is disturbance of the hormonal system. The hormone, it seems, causes a shift of fatty matter which is then deposited in out of the way areas of the body, and results in dilation of the blood vessels. This allows the build-up of fluid, toxins and fat in the connective tissues and also results in poor circulation – another cause of cellulite, as we have seen.

REMOVING CELLULITE

There are two main elements to cellulite removal: the first is to make sure all excess toxins and fluids are eliminated from fat cells, and the second is to try and restore the connective tissues to their former condition, to prevent recurrence of the condition.

The Elancyl range of products contain ivy extract, butcherbroom to improve venous circulation and reduce the amount of fluid released into the tissues, and matein, from the mate tree in South America. This works to break down cellulite nodules and allows them to be eliminated via the circulation. Vitamin E is used to zap the free radicals – excess oxygen molecules which can harm the immune system and cause disease.

These ingredients are contained in the famous green Elancyl glove (who hasn't at some time had one of these at the end of their bath?) which enables the ingredients to be massaged in. To be effective, the glove has to be used for five minutes daily, for at least a month. It doesn't do any good just sitting at the end of the bath! Recent tests in France on the glove method found that cellulite disappeared dramatically with one month's continual use according to the instructions.

Clinical results using the MP24 (twenty-four hours slow release) method, where 'microparticles' are massaged daily into the skin without the use of the glove, found that improvement was noticed between the eighth and fifteenth day in 90 per cent of cases, and only 10 per cent of cases took more than fifteen days to show distinct signs of improvement. The doctors in France who carried out the surveys, using the Elancyl products, were satisfied that there was a dramatic improvement. For this particular research, subjects did not resort to any other means of reducing cellulite, such as stringent dieting or exercise.

At this point the cynics among you might say: well, of course the manufacturers are going to say that their product works. Would they seriously publish research saying it *didn't* work unless they wanted to go out of business? So the proof of the pudding has to be in the eating; I decided to try Elancyl for myself, religiously, for a month, to see whether the products made any difference whatever. I had, admittedly, already got rid of 90 per cent of my cellulite by the aromatherapy method, but as it had been there for about 20 years there were still some stubborn areas deep down. I used the Elancyl product specially recommended for stubborn cellulite, or *zones rebelles* as they say in France.

When I went for my next aromatherapy, my therapist said I was in 'very good shape' – even though I had not been for an aromatherapy massage for several months. Even more cellulite, she said, had disappeared since the last time.

I have somewhat revised my opinion of patent creams since the original edition of this book appeared – mainly because I know so much more about cellulite than I did when I started. *But I will only believe the claims of patent products where these are backed up by serious research carried out in hospitals by proper, independent doctors – and have published papers on their results.* There are now so many anti-cellulite preparations on the market; most of these are riding on the backs of the companies who have carried out proper research, and have investigated the subject seriously. Yet most companies manufacturing anti-cellulite treatments have not carried out their own proper research into the subject.

I now believe that some patent creams can work – so long as the massage is kept up daily for at least a month. I also believe that the expensive creams work better *after* the cellulite has been attacked by aromatherapy, and if possible, professional lymphatic drainage massage. Also, there is the diet – don't forget that. It is most important, and means that the cellulite has at least a chance of disappearing for ever. There can only be, at best, a modest difference when creams and lotions are applied, and there is no attempt made to follow the anti-cellulite diet.

Even after most of the cellulite has gone, most people still need a certain amount of maintenance. The problem will tend to come back if you let it because once you have established a tendency towards cellulite, that tendency will always be there.

But how will you know whether your patent cream is working? By the same method as the aromatherapy oils; taking measurements and noting the frequency of urination. When cellulite starts to shift, the very first thing you notice is that you want to pee every hour on the hour. The other unmistakable sign is that bulges and indentations start to smooth out and also you lose that cold, clammy feeling.

It is, though, notoriously difficult to know for sure whether such and such a heavily-advertised cream might be working, or whether one is being over-optimistic or influenced by wishful thinking. Beauty and health magazines which ask readers to be guinea pigs and try certain treatments for a month or so find that the reports back are rarely positive. Readers almost always say that the products have made no difference whatever and that their lumps and bulges are as firmly in place as ever. *Which?* magazine recently tested a whole series of patent anti-cellulite products to see whether they made any difference. They also asked a number of volunteers to test cheap creams – the thing about most anti-cellulite products is that they are extremely expensive.

The *Which?* researchers came to the conclusion that the cheap creams worked just as well as the expensive imported products BUT – and this is an important but – they came to the conclusion that daily application and dedicated massage does indeed make a difference. Cellulite deposits definitely disappeared with diligent, regular massage. This tends to confirm what Dr Terence Ryan found that massage is the best way to treat the problem.

Although there are very many creams on the market now, with more coming out all the time, it is far better to use essential oils than creams, as they penetrate deeper down into the skin and have an effect on the whole system. For thousands of years, Indian ayurvedic medicine has known that herbal oils have a dramatic detoxifying effect, something that not even the most expensive cream can achieve.

As Frances Clifford says, you can't stop essential oils from working, whereas creams will stay on the surface.

WARNING: do not use essential oils in conjunction with sunbathing, if you are planning a pregnancy, or during lactation. It is good to sweat when on an anti-cellulite programme, as part of the detoxification process, and steam rooms in health clubs or at health farms give a nice wet heat. Saunas may be too dehydrating and, in any case, always check with your doctor before using a sauna treatment.

Remember, though, that whatever you do, not everybody in the world will have pin-thin, rock-hard, super-smooth thighs. Although every woman in the modern world may want these, it's just not humanly possible, given the huge variety of shapes and sizes we come in. All we can say is that cellulite is an aberration, a disorder, and it can be made to disappear, with enough dedication. But once it goes, not everybody will have the wonder thighs they might like. There will still be some women with inherited fatter thighs than others – unfortunately.

ARE THERE DIFFERENT TYPES OF CELLULITE?

Recently, researchers have identified two distinct types of cellulite: the type that sits on the surface and the 'stubborn' cellulite which is much further down, and which takes far more effort to encourage to disappear. I certainly found that when my 'surface' cellulite disappeared, the 'stubborn' stuff further down became much more in evidence, and that this was far harder to shift.

Sally Gilbert Wilson is a skin specialist who has been working with clients in her Harley Street practice for over thirty years. She has recently turned her attention to treating cellulite, and believes that nowadays, we can categorize it in several ways.

There is, she believes, the predominately DIETARY kind of cellulite, which is associated with a high-fat diet. This type of cellulite is easy to cure because it responds well to the anti-cellulite diet.

The METABOLIC type of cellulite is common in slim people, and is caused mainly by sluggish metabolism and a sedentary job. Skin brushing to detoxify and the anti-cellulite diet are usually enough to shift toxic matter caused in this way.

The mainly HORMONAL kind of cellulite is found on women who suffer from PMT, post-natal depression or who have problems with the pill. Deep connective tissue massage is the best solution here, Sally believes.

According to Sally, the worst kind of cellulite, and the hardest to shift is the INHERITED kind. If your sisters, mother, grandmother or other female relatives suffered from cellulite, then do not exactly abandon hope – but expect the struggle to be a prolonged one. My own problem was mainly an inherited one, which is why my cellulite was so difficult to remove. However, aromatherapy combined with skin brushing to improve circulation provided the best form of attack.

The strangest explanation I have heard to explain why some people suffer from inherited cellulite is that it constitutes excess baggage – negative thoughts and bad karma – from a previous life. American past-life therapist Denise Linn, who gives lectures on cellulite, believes that the toxic wastes are formed mainly by negative habits ingrained from previous lives. Past-life therapy, she believes, can help us to understand why we are carrying these deposits, and then release and yield them up.

I'm not sure about this explanation, which is certainly the crankiest I have heard so far – but then I remind myself that, 10 years ago, every doctor was laughing the idea of 'toxins' to scorn. Now, few doctors dismiss the possibility that many systems may be holding and accumulating waste matter they are unable to eliminate through the normal eliminative channels. So, perhaps in 10 years' time, the 'past life' explanation of cellulite will no longer seem so strange. And, if Denise Linn's treatment gets rid of the offending lumps and bumps, well – who's to say she's talking rubbish?

The one serious flaw in her argument, of course, is that only women get cellulite. Why don't men carry excess baggage on their thighs from past lives? Surely women can't be singled out for this bizarre punishment?

OTHER FORMS OF TREATMENT

A form of treatment which has become popular in France, although it has hardly caught on in the UK yet, is *mesotherapy*, where cellulite-laden areas are pricked with a series of tiny needles which penetrate the area with anti-cellulite oils. Apparently, it doesn't hurt, and it should certainly work.

NORMAFORM

This is a form of lymphatic drainage pioneered by Dr Denis Melrose of Hammersmith Hospital, West London. He and his team designed pressure therapy leggings for the use of hospital patients to minimize the risk of pulmonary embolism during surgical operations. After being in use at Hammersmith for about fifteen years, the equipment has now been redesigned for use in health and beauty salons and health farms. Basically, the equipment consists of a pair of inflatable leggings which look rather like enormous Wellington boots. The leggings are inflated to fit the legs very tightly, and constitute a form of massage. The air pressure is designed to improve the natural circulation of the blood and tissue fluids through stimulation of the lymph flow. The idea is that the treatment will rid the body of water retention.

The treatment is quite painless, although it feels rather strange, and after about an hour's treatment, when the leggings are taken off, you will notice a network of tiny white lines up and down your legs. This is where the lymph channels have been raised, and the lines will go down in about an hour. No harm results from this treatment.

According to Professor Melrose, the equipment works to speed up the flow of lymph in much the same way as vigorous exercise, and helps to rid tissues of waste products. Excess water in the tissues, adds

Professor Melrose, means an inefficient waste disposal system which can, in time, lead to actual ill health. About six treatments would be necessary to rid the legs of cellulite deposits. Again, this form of treatment is best combined with the diet outlined earlier, otherwise the cellulite will just come back.

Note: There is *no* way of escaping the diet! All expensive creams and patent treatments, plus visits to a beauty therapist, will certainly help, but around 60 per cent of the effort has to come from *you*! In spite of ever-more sophisticated treatments to separate you from your cellulite (and your money), nothing will work in the long-term unless you are prepared to adhere to the diet.

Most health farms and beauty clinics now offer a whole range of passive treatments for cellulite, such as ionotheremie – thermal clay treatments where you are smeared with a thick green substance then an electrical current embeds the active ingredients deep into the tissues – and toning tables designed to give you isometric exercises. The trouble with these is that one application, or even treatments over the period of a week, won't make the slightest bit of difference. Many people book themselves in for a week at a health farm and are then disappointed because in spite of starving, having loads of treatments and electrical currents passed through them, fierce water jets applied to the legs and so on, the cellulite is just as firmly in place at the end of the stay.

This doesn't mean the treatments are no good. A week simply isn't long enough to make any noticeable difference to the cellulite deposits. Few people are aware of any improvement before a period of a month, at least.

FASTING

In common with most self-indulgent people, I found the anti-cellulite diet extremely difficult. It is not easy to deny yourself all your favourite foods and drinks, and the days seem long indeed without frequent punctuations of tea, coffee, cigarettes and wine – or whatever your particular vice is.

I can't suggest any easy way of accustoming yourself to the anti-cellulite diet, except to stress that it is absolutely necessary for anybody who is serious about losing their toxic wastes. But I can recommend fasting as a way of providing a short break from food and mood-altering drinks, and to help you get to know your body better.

If dieting is difficult, then fasting is even more so. But an increasing number of doctors now believe that a short fast can be the quickest and most effective way of ridding the body of toxic deposits, of improving circulation and aiding the digestive system. And if you can join a fasting weekend, where you are united in misery with like-minded mortals, then it can even become quite an enjoyable activity. Fasting is also an excellent way to break links with habits, such as smoking or an over-indulgence in caffeine. Also, after the fast, you simply won't want to eat rich, saturated-fat foods for a time, so it is also a way of getting used to eating salads and fresh vegetables, rather than stuffing yourself with cream cakes and junk foods.

I have found that fasting definitely helps to speed up the detoxifying process – and also gives a positive outlook which may be difficult to achieve with dieting alone. As I suspected I would not have the self-discipline to fast on my own, I joined a residential weekend run by the Sivananda Yoga Centre, in Putney, London, where you eat nothing and drink nothing but herb tea and mineral water for two and a half days.

We all gathered together at six o'clock on Friday evening, having eaten nothing since lunch. We were advised to eat a very light lunch, and not to stuff ourselves against the coming famine. One 'must' for fasters is to keep physically active and half an hour after we arrived, and settled ourselves into our makeshift dormitory accommodation, we did an hour-and-a-half's yoga exercises. Dr Peter Mansfield, a British GP who is a keen advocate of short fasts, believes that physical activity is essential to a successful fast. If you hibernate and crawl into a corner, he says, you are encouraging the toxins to stay in the system. The combination of fasting and exercise helps them to dissipate fast.

After the yoga, we had an introductory talk and introduction, then (as it was a meditation centre) we also joined in the meditation and chanting. Some of the participants found this rather odd, and unsettling. My own view is that the chanting and meditation takes your mind off food – it's better to do something than nothing. And an unusual activity such as chanting is one which for most people does not have any connotations with eating, unlike sitting in front of the telly watching a video.

Most of us felt fairly well on the Friday night, although some slept only fitfully. We were woken up at 5.30 a.m. the next morning for more chanting and meditation before the next yoga class at 8. Mineral water and herb tea were always available, and you are advised to drink as much as possible, to flush out the system. By about 10 o'clock on Saturday morning some of us were feeling slightly weak and queasy, and some had developed bad headaches – a sure sign that the fasting is working. We all went for a long walk and then had a rest before the afternoon session of talks, yoga, more chanting and meditation. By mid-afternoon, some of us were feeling distinctly grumpy and bad-tempered. Also even the most voluble of us went strangely quiet. Some felt shivery and cold.

We watched a 'spiritual' video on the Saturday evening, and went to bed early. Some people vomited throughout the night, others were overwhelmed by the strangeness of it all. There were complaints about the showers, the cramped accommodation, the weirdness of the chanting. But really, everybody was having to come to terms with not eating. The time seemed endless.

By Sunday, most of us had gone extremely quiet and withdrawn, although the bad headaches and the nauseous feelings were beginning to pass. There was more yoga, more long walks, more chanting and meditation, more talks about diet and nutrition – and then, at 8.30, at last, we had some food: stewed apples, which are now seen as the best way to break a fast. At this stage, we were advised on how to break the fast over the following few days – fruit only for the first day, fresh vegetables for the second and then gradually introducing grains and wholemeal bread. We met again on Thursday evening at the Centre for a celebration meal, and compared notes. Without exception, everybody had felt light and positive – and far better in health for the experience.

After taking part now in several fasting weekends, I would highly recommend this way of getting started on a completely different diet. As the fasting is carried out under supervision, by people who are extremely experienced, there is no danger at all, even if you start to feel ill during the fast. As a general rule, the more toxic your system, the more ill you will feel. This is especially noticeable with meat eaters. The healthier your diet, the less you will suffer during the actual weekend.

My own view is that fasting is far easier on a residential weekend such as I attended (and needless to say, it's far cheaper) than going to a health farm, where only some of the clients may be fasting. Also, the contrast between the sybaritic surroundings and your deprivation at a health farm may be almost unbearable.

If you find the anti-cellulite diet particularly difficult, do consider fasting as a way in. You will feel so pleased with yourself that you are encouraged to continue – completing a fast gives a tremendous feeling of achievement – and your body will feel so light and healthy that you will be far less inclined to stuff it with rubbish. But, like anything else, good intentions start to fade when you are back in the outside world . So, for anybody who is serious about keeping cellulite off, I would recommend going on two or three fasting weekends a year, if possible. Apart from the health benefits, there is also spiritual uplift to be gained from not eating: people find they gain valuable insights into themselves when the anaesthetic effect of food is removed for a few days. Fasting is, of course, the most ancient way of attaining self-knowledge.

Never believe that cellulite is a trivial problem! Because it has been so closely aligned with the beauty industry, which has never had a good name anyway, cellulite has been rather dismissed as something for vain, empty-minded people to worry about. But changing your diet, changing your shape, having a different and more confident outlook are never trivial matters. Cellulite ladens one – mentally and emotionally as well as physically. Without it, you'll feel lighter, more confident, a more worthwhile person. Speaking from experience, this is not an exaggeration.

Now that cellulite is at last being taken seriously by the medical profession, and being investigated with highly sophisticated machinery, perhaps the next decade will bring about even more effective treatments for this condition. Having been identified – with scorn and jeering – by the cosmetic and alternative medicine professions, cellulite is at last being accepted as a genuine, distressing complaint, even if it is hardly life-threatening or seriously injurious to health.

Cellulite is injurious to self-esteem and body image, and these days, when so much flesh is being exposed all the time and nobody wants to become noticeably old, it must be taken seriously.

PART II
THE ANTI-CELLULITE DIET

Chapter 9

The Importance of Diet

Since *How to Banish Cellulite Forever* first appeared, a lot of patent anti-cellulite treatments have come on to the market. The anti-cellulite business appears to be getting bigger all the time. Most of the new treatments have been brought out by major, multi-national cosmetic houses and introduced with huge amounts of hype and enormous advertising budgets. The treatments promise that diligent application will deliver smooth, bulge-free contours, and this message is underlined by pictures of super-slim models displaying impossibly thin thighs.

True, the word 'cellulite' is rarely mentioned when these products are advertised. 'Cellulite' is a word that is still not officially admitted in respectable cosmetic or medical circles. We hear instead terms like 'body sculpturing' and 'contouring' – the advertisements are very clever indeed.

Most of these creams and lotions containing the results of the 'latest scientific research' are extremely expensive. But do they work? Well, *very* diligent and dedicated long-term use may make some small difference but the truth is that no anti-cellulite cream, lotion or oil can have very much effect unless you are prepared to undertake the anti-cellulite diet as well. Otherwise, as fast as you are sculpturing your body with the aid of the scientifically developed cream you are encouraging new bulges and bumps to form by eating the wrong food. So you will be fighting a guaranteed losing battle.

I am not suggesting that diet is the *only* way to deal with cellulite – indeed, in *How to Banish Cellulite Forever* I explained at length that for most people a fourfold attack is essential. Not only diet, but body brushing, aromatherapy and massage are needed to encourage the body to yield up its long-held cellulite deposits. But an effective anti-cellulite regime must start with diet in order to attack the problem from the inside out rather than the outside in.

It used to be believed that the skin was a completely waterproof covering which nothing could penetrate. We now know that this is not the case, and a whole new range of cosmetics and transdermal drugs – where a patch is applied to the skin and the drug seeps through to the area beneath – has been developed which take advantage of this new finding. Also, the growing popularity of research into essential oils has shown that certain substances applied to the skin can have a definite therapeutic effect on the whole body. A number of NHS hospitals in Britain are now using the science of essential oils for treating chronic and severe pain – with excellent results.

Aromatherapy is of proven value in the fight against cellulite, but it can never be the whole answer. In order to rid yourself of cellulite deposits you have to employ both strategies – diet and aromatherapy – and both require quite a lot of hard work.

Any reputable aromatherapist will tell you that at least sixty per cent of the effort must come from you, and the most important part of that effort comes with the diet. If you are serious about banishing cellulite forever you must stay on the diet for the rest of your life. Of course, the very rigorous initial regime does not have to be kept up – nor should it, as it does not constitute a long-term balanced diet – but it is important to develop a diet for life that will maintain the body in a detoxified and toned-up condition.

The reason for this is that cellulite is always liable to come back, much as dust is always trying to settle on household objects, and tarnish on silver and brass. You can only keep it away by constant vigilance. That is an uncomfortable but true fact of life about cellulite. Cellulite describes fat cells that have become filled with waterlogged toxic deposits, and it is very stubborn stuff indeed. In fact, it can be so very difficult to get rid of that many fat and obesity experts have declared that it is impossible. They tell us that we just have to accept these awful lumps and bumps as part of being a woman.

That's what I did for twenty years – just assumed that the hard, lumpy deposits were as much a part of me as my ears and eyes. Now that I have straight, bulge-free thighs for the first time in my adult life I know that cellulite is not an inescapable aspect of being a woman but an aberration, something abnormal, something that should not be there.

Nobody should ever feel discouraged. It is perfectly possible to shift cellulite, however long it has been there, if you make up your mind to pay scrupulous attention to your diet. It is now increasingly realized by doctors and scientists that diet plays a far larger part in all aspects of health maintenance than was previously believed. For many years, doctors laughed at the idea that illness could be caused or made worse by diet, and they insisted on telling us that nowadays everybody ate a perfectly balanced, nutritious diet, at least in the West. Those people who suspected that diet might be at the root of their health problems were usually written off as time-wasters and hypochondriacs. Alternative practitioners who tried to treat illnesses by dietary means were dismissed as charlatans and unqualified get-rich-quick merchants.

Now, however, the situation has changed beyond all recognition. Orthodox medical opinion is fast coming round to the view that diet may be a contributory factor to a wide variety of chronic conditions, from arthritis and heart disease to cancer, ME, multiple sclerosis, allergies, asthma, eczema, hyperactivity in children, migraine, irritable bowel syndrome, ulcers, skin disorders, candida albicans, low energy levels, and infertility.

There is increasing evidence that food intolerance is a very real problem, and may be responsible for a wide range of illnesses. It seems that everyday foods such as milk, wheat and sugar could be at the root of poor health in many cases. Allergies, particularly food allergies, are becoming more common all the time, and doctors are having great success in both diagnosing and treating a large number of allergy complaints by diet.

Most people consider that cellulite is not a serious illness. In fact, it is usually not considered an illness at all, and concern over cellulite is often seen as an expression of vanity. With so many problems in the world, how dare women worry about a few lumps and bumps? I am sure one of the reasons so many people – including women – deny the existence of cellulite is that there is a guilty feeling that it is wrong to be so concerned about appearance. After all, even if you have cellulite, you probably do not actually feel unwell from it. And if you are dismayed by the sight of your naked body, well, you just have a negative body image which must be overcome by positive thinking. There is a school of thought that says women should be happy with their bodies whatever shape they are, and should not put themselves at the mercy of cosmetic houses and questionable practitioners who have identified yet another area of women's bodies to worry about. This line of thought says that our present obsession with slimness and eternal youth is media-led, so much nonsense, and that 'real' women have lumps, bumps, wrinkles, grey hair and uneven teeth, so we should not all try to look the same, or attempt to conform to an impossible ideal.

To some extent I go along with these arguments. There is no reason why we should all be exactly the same shape and size, production-line women. We are all made differently, and not everybody is going to be five feet ten and size eight, whatever self-tortures are applied.

However, I also believe that it is easier to love oneself and have a positive body image when one has done one's very best to maintain one's optimum shape and condition. To worry about cellulite is not the same as worrying about a big nose, or thick ankles – it is not merely a cosmetic concern but an actual health problem. I am now convinced of this. Furthermore, although the presence of cellulite may not exactly make you feel ill, you will certainly feel a great deal better about yourself when it has gone. There is no doubt in my mind that my general health improved along with my appearance once I decided to mount a concerted attack on cellulite.

At the same time as my cellulite gradually disappeared – and it took about three months in my case before a real effect was visible – I noticed that I had new energy levels, that I could walk much further without getting tired, and that I felt generally cleaner and less clogged-up inside. So many of us have become used to a less-than-optimum health and energy level that we accept it as normal.

While using myself as a guinea pig I learned a lot about health and nutrition and how my body worked. Before, I had hardly taken any interest, and had just fed it at intervals. Now I am extremely careful about what I eat. My whole system has become more sensitively tuned, and I have started to imagine what might be going on in my body when I have alcohol, butter-covered pasta, coffee and ice-cream all in the same meal. Although this combination is delicious when you are eating it, you don't feel so good afterwards. On the anti-cellulite diet, you will feel good all the time. Added bonuses are that the condition of your skin and hair will improve and you will experience a whole new positive feeling about yourself. Most cellulite sufferers do not feel in the least bit ill – at least not because of their cellulite, because the body has done its very best to transfer toxic wastes to out-of-the-way areas where they will do least harm. But the very existence of cellulite is an indication that not everything is well inside. It is a warning that your body is taking in more waste matter than it can comfortably handle, and that your circulation is sluggish.

Once you start the diet everything speeds up simultaneously. You will notice that transit time – the amount of time food takes to go through the digestive tract and be eliminated from your body – gets faster and that your head feels much clearer.

The anti-cellulite diet is important because it gives the body a chance to detoxify itself so that the cellulite can be eliminated. The reason it has accumulated in the first place is that the body's organs of elimination have too much work to do. The only way to detoxify your body is to eat as many pure, natural substances as possible and cut out all the refined, processed, non-nutritive foods. This gives the lymphatic system – the body's own vacuum cleaner – an opportunity to do its job properly and dispose of toxic substances.

Since my first book on cellulite was published, many people who do not wish to relinquish their bad eating habits have informed me that this or that person eats nothing but Mars bars, gets through thirty cigarettes and a bottle of wine a day, and still has no cellulite. People have told me that most dancers and athletes, some of whom eat a terrible junk-food diet, have not a trace of cellulite.

Well, so they might. And if you haven't got any cellulite, then you can continue eating all the rubbish you like. But if you have, and you wish to get rid of it, you have no choice but to follow the diet. If you have cellulite, and have had it for a long time, you are not going to lose it on a diet of chips, sausages, ice-cream, chocolate, cigarettes and alcohol.

Dancers and athletes do not have cellulite because even though they may eat a terrible diet they are on the move all the time and exercise strenuously. Cellulite does not have a chance to form on them. But these same people often succumb to arthritis in later life, and this is very likely closely connected with the bad diet they ate when in training.

The problem is, the vast majority of women who suffer from cellulite are couch potatoes – as well as eating self-indulgently, they never take any exercise. This was me for twenty years. I have always been a greedy pig over food, and at the same time physically lazy. I smoked and drank and took the contraceptive pill throughout my twenties. I hated exercise, I couldn't bear the thought of Spartan eating regimes. I shared the attitude of Milton's *Comus*

... if all the world
should in a pet of temperance feed on pulse
Drink the clear stream and nothing wear but frieze,
The all-Giver would be unthanked, would be unpraised,
Not half his riches known and yet despised ...

Now I have a different attitude. I believe that if all the world did feed on pulses (a wonderful anti-cellulite food, and also good for unfurring the arteries) and drank the clear, unpolluted stream, the world's health would improve enormously and very many of our 'diseases of civilization', as author Brian Inglis has called them, would disappear – including cellulite.

The relationship of diet to cellulite means that the worse the diet, the higher the risk of cellulite deposits. Not everybody who smokes fifty cigarettes a day will die of lung cancer, but they are at high risk. The same with cellulite. The more junk you put in your system, the higher the risk of cellulite will be. You may not succumb – but your chances are not good.

If you have cellulite – and around eighty per cent of Western women have – then it will have been encouraged to form by a combination of a toxic diet, sedentary habits causing poor circulation, and taking in more pollutants of all kinds than your body can comfortably handle. There is also a hereditary factor in cellulite – if your mother has it then your chances of getting it will be high.

Modern processed foods encourage cellulite deposits because the body is not equipped to deal with artificial colours, flavours, pesticides, hormones from dairy produce, and large amounts of refined sugar. So it rebels, in one way or another. One woman may have terrible headaches, while another has cellulite. Men develop beer bellies and suffer heart attacks. Children often become hyperactive. Nobody is immune from the bad effects of an unhealthy diet, and there are many ways that ill health of one sort or another may manifest itself.

Even if we eat a highly nutritious diet we still take in waste products and toxic matter. But if the diet is basically pure and natural the digestive system will be able to cope with any rubbish, sending it to the organs of elimination (the skin, bowels, kidneys and lymphatic system) to be passed out of the body. To facilitate this, the colon contains bacteria which work to break down food particles into a form that can be processed. However, if there is not enough beneficial bacteria in the colon, waste matter becomes re-absorbed into the bloodstream where it can cause a variety of conditions. In women, although not in men, the female hormone oestrogen does its best to make sure these toxic wastes do not go anywhere near vital organs in the event of a pregnancy. So it sends them to the thighs, hips, buttocks and upper arms.

The trouble is, beneficial bacteria are easily killed off by many aspects of modern living, such as antibiotics, high fat and heavy protein diets, high sugar consumption and too little dietary fibre. The anti-cellulite diet, however, will encourage the body's eco-system to return to normal and to eliminate waste matter effectively.

The main purpose of the anti-cellulite diet is to enable the body to detoxify itself by eliminating long-held wastes. It is not a reducing diet as such, although if you are overweight as well it will certainly help you get your weight back to normal.

I cannot overstress the importance of the right diet in an effective anti-cellulite regime. When I first embarked on the programme myself I was highly sceptical and also, if the truth be told, extremely reluctant to give up all the foods I enjoyed – rich cheesecakes, cheesy moussakas, buttery pasta dishes. All these foods are described by nutritionists as 'highly palatable', as they deliver a feeling of fullness and satisfaction. But they don't always do such nice things to your innards. While you are giving your taste buds short-term satisfaction you may be being unkind to your body.

Many women imagine that crinkly, bumpy skin is inevitable as they grow older. But although skin and contours cannot indefinitely keep the smooth, wrinkle-free appearance of youth, cellulite need never be a problem. It's ageing, unsightly and unhealthy, and your outward sign of a sluggish system. Embark on the anti-cellulite diet and you are half-way towards getting rid of it.

Chapter 10

The Principles Behind the Diet

The basic idea behind the anti-cellulite diet is that it is high in nutritional value and low in all substances that can cause physical degeneration, addictions, cravings and toxic conditions within the body. So it is an extremely healthy diet in any case. You will feel much better on this diet than on the standard modern intake of processed and overcooked foods.

It has recently been said that everybody now knows they should eat more fruit and vegetables, less sugar, fat, particularly animal fats, and drink less coffee and alcohol. However, being aware of what a healthy diet consists of is another matter from actually eating healthily. A recent (1989) survey by the market research firm Taylor Nelson found that the diet of the average British schoolchild is worse than ever, with *fewer* fresh fruits and vegetables being eaten than ten years ago. The diet of the average adult is hardly better; we still do not eat enough fruit and vegetables, and we still rely too much on convenience foods and instant taste sensations. Convenience foods are the nutritional equivalent of a romantic novel, which may be enjoyable and escapist when you are reading it, but is by no means Good Literature. Chocolate bars and ice-cream are escapist food, delivering only calories and little nutritional value.

The diet recommended in this book has the opposite effect – it feeds and nourishes the body properly. It is the Shakespeare, rather than the Barbara Cartland – of diets, perhaps harder work to start with, but ultimately much more rewarding and enjoyable.

For the ultimate in nutrition, your raw materials should be organically grown. A few years ago it would have been pointless to recommend organic foods, as these were extremely expensive and difficult to obtain. Now, however, more supermarkets are specializing in organically grown produce, and the space given over to wholefoods is getting bigger all the time. It has become easy to follow the anti-cellulite diet, and inexpensive as well. The recipes in this book all work out far cheaper than frozen and convenience foods.

And what do they taste like? After all, if the diet doesn't taste good, nobody will stick to it, especially when there is such an abundant choice of more tempting products easily available. When I was testing the recipes I realized that I could not rely simply on my own judgment, so I invited a selection of people to come and try them. They were all pronounced absolutely delicious, even by large men who had no cellulite and never would have any, but who did have vast appetites.

It is basically a matter of retraining your taste buds to enjoy good food instead of nutritionally empty food. As with anything else, it is all too easy to develop lazy, bad habits and all too difficult to inculcate good ones. Substituting good for bad ingrained habits is hard, and requires constant practice. At first, I found that sticking to the diet needed attention, as well as motivation. If I wasn't thinking about it, I could easily slip back into my old ways. The only answer was to make the diet a way of life, which is what it has become.

I can now honestly say that I prefer my anti-cellulite diet – which I no longer regard as specifically anti-cellulite, but protective against all degenerative diseases – to the one I was eating before, and that there have been very many bonuses apart from the loss of the hideous orange-peel flesh.

My skin is softer and more wrinkle-free, my hair remains in good condition even though I now punish it with perms and colours, and my general health remains absolutely A1. When I recently had a medical – my first for over twenty years – the doctor could find nothing wrong with me at all.

I cannot be sure what the exact relation is between my good health and what I eat. What I can say, though, is that my contemporaries who do not eat a good diet are not as healthy or in such good shape. On the other hand, just about everybody I know who does eat a good diet – and really, there aren't all that many of us, not even with the proliferation of diet and health books currently on the market – are in superb shape, men as well. Apart from anything else, a bad diet has an ageing effect. Smoking, drinking and junk foods all accelerate the ageing process mightily, especially past the age of thirty-five.

The anti-cellulite diet detoxifies, purifies, and keeps your innards clean and free from waste matter. And that cannot be bad.

Chapter 11

Is It Healthy? Is It Well-Balanced?

You should not imagine that the anti-cellulite diet is suitable only for those who wish to be rid of the lumps and bumps on their thighs. It is a healthy diet that will benefit everybody who eats it. Although it will very definitely help cellulite to disperse, this is not the only good thing about the diet. It will also give the best possible nutritional protection against ill health and those chronic conditions that are now considered to have a dietary ingredient. Studies in the United States have shown categorically that those on a low-fat, high-fibre diet have far lower incidences of all degenerative diseases than people who eat junk food. The nutrition plan detailed in this book will help hyperactive children, people with allergies, women suffering from PMT, and people who succumb to frequent headaches, anxiety attacks or irritable bowel syndrome. It will also help to protect against heart attacks, cancer and arthritis.

But is it well-balanced? Does it contain enough protein, fats and carbohydrates? The answer is emphatically yes. Whenever people are recommended a low-fat, low-protein intake, they always ask the same question: will I get enough protein?

Strangely enough, nobody ever asks whether a diet of burgers or fried chicken will give them enough of the nutrients they need. I've found that people can even feel nervous of changing to a healthy diet because of what their neighbours or friends might think. They say they don't want to be labelled among the brown-rice-and-sandals brigade. Since the 'green' craze, however, this attitude is mercifully disappearing, even among the worst dietary diehards.

In the West, there is no danger whatever of anybody going short of protein or fat. In fact, most people eat far too much of both, with disastrous consequences for their health. Most of us have grown up with the idea that protein is the most important dietary requirement, and that this is mainly supplied in the form of meat, fish, and dairy products such as eggs and cheese. In fact, anti-cellulite recipes exclude these items wherever possible. You will not find a single egg or cheese recipe in the whole book, except for a few instances where low-fat cheeses such as cottage cheese or quark are recommended.

Most of us have heard that meat and fish provide first-class protein whereas vegetable products provide only a second-class version. Therefore, people wonder, how do vegetarians make up this deficiency?

Proteins consist of long chains of amino acids, chemicals that are vital for body growth, maintenance and repair. Some amino acids are 'essential' and can only be supplied through the diet. Most meats and fish provide all the essential amino acids required, whereas vegetable products do not. Foods that deliver the eight essential amino acids are known as complete proteins, whereas foods that provide only some are known as incomplete proteins. Vegetable products are incomplete proteins.

But that does not mean you cannot obtain all your protein requirements from plant foods alone. You can, so long as you make sure you have enough variety. A dish of brown rice and beans will make a complete protein, as together these foods deliver all of the eight essential amino acids. Nuts and rice, or nuts and vegetables together, also make up a complete protein. Baked beans on wholemeal toast are a complete protein.

Most modern slimming diets are low in fat, and some do not have any fat in them at all. However, although most of us in the West eat far too much fat – around forty per cent of the average adult diet consists of fat – we do need some. Fats are necessary for energy, for protection against many diseases and for the synthesis of essential chemicals and hormones in the body. A certain amount of fat is also required for smooth skin, shining hair and strong nails. So the anti-cellulite diet is by no means fat-free.

Yet there is no butter or margarine in any of the recipes. The reason for this is our old enemies, free radicals. When vegetables or meats are fried in fat, huge amounts of free radicals tend to be released. Also, when cooking in oil or fat, you are probably taking in more fat than you realize. We can obtain all the fat we need from unsalted nuts, avocados, and salad dressings made from extra-virgin cold-pressed olive oil. Many of the recipes in this book use oil for dips and dressings, but the fats are not cooked or heated.

The fats used in the anti-cellulite diet are mono-unsaturated, which means they are unlikely to release free radicals into the system. I do not want to enter into a butter-versus-margarine debate here, except to say that, as a general rule, I favour the foods that have been around for thousands of years and have had time to prove themselves, rather than modern laboratory concoctions that contain artificial ingredients. I would rather use small amounts of butter than margarine, and olive oil rather than anonymous 'vegetable' oils which may have been highly processed. My guideline is: the closer to nature, the better. Butter itself is not a highly processed food, although I am wary of it to some extent because the cows may have been fed on all sorts of hormones and antibiotics, and the milk itself will probably have been treated and pasteurized. Cold-pressed olive oil, dark green in colour and with a satisfying sediment at the bottom, has simply been pressed from the raw material – olives – and is as near to nature as any fat can be.

I used to be a real butter and cream freak. Now, I hardly ever buy butter, and instead I use sesame seed and sunflower seed spreads. If you have children, try giving them natural, unsalted, untreated peanut butter without colourings or additives. All children like it, and it is better for them than butter. Instead of buying double or clotted cream, which I used to delight in, I now make my own nut creams with cashews or almonds, liquidized with water, a little honey and natural vanilla essence. They are wonderful – and go down a treat with visitors.

No one actually needs animal fats, in any shape or form. They are all highly saturated, which means in technical terms that the bonds between the carbon atoms that make up the fat are saturated with hydrogen atoms. These fats are not essential for health or nutrition in any way, although polyunsaturated and monounsaturated fats are. Many fats needed by the body can be made up from other foods, such as complex carbohydrates. One reason the anti-cellulite diet contains hardly any meat is because up to eighty per cent of the calories in many meats are derived from fat. Pork and beef are the most fat-laden, and even eggs are sixty-six per cent fat.

The other main macronutrient, carbohydrate, is also essential for health. In the old days, slimming diets were low in carbohydrates, and recommended minimal intakes of potatoes, bread, pasta and rice. We now have a different approach and believe that complex carbohydrates – that is, carbohydrates derived from whole sources – are an essential nutrient. Complex carbohydrates, which contain sugars in a chemically complex form, are better than simple, or refined, carbohydrates such as white sugar, because they are slow-release foods, making them a good source of stamina and continued energy.

The more you cook carbohydrate-rich foods, the more chance there is of the starch content being broken down, so that the sugar enters the blood stream too quickly. Complex carbohydrates are also a good source of fibre, which is essential for the quick transit of food through the digestive system.

There are two main kinds of fibre, soluble and insoluble. Wheat and wheat products are mainly composed of insoluble fibre, whereas oat products consist of the soluble kind. This means they have a greater ability to absorb and help to eliminate waste matter. So wherever possible you should eat oat cereals in preference to wheat-based ones, and unsweetened oatcakes rather than biscuits or bread. Oat germ and oat bran can be sprinkled on soups or cereals instead of wheat bran.

Does the anti-cellulite diet provide enough vitamins and minerals? Yes, it does. I take no supplements of any kind and have been perfectly healthy for very many years without needing vitamin or mineral pills. There is some evidence that without meat you may go short of vitamin B12, which is hard to find in sufficient quantity in vegetable products. However, some nutritionists say that the body seems easily able to make up the deficiency without any problem. In any case, the main health risk from the standard diet now eaten in the West is not malnutrition from undereating but from eating too much of the wrong food.

I can already hear another objection. But isn't this diet boring and tedious? Won't you get awfully tired of it? No, not at all. Since you have to try harder to make the meals interesting, you actually get more variety than on a standard meat-and-two-vegetables diet. Also, the meals are far tastier. After all, what could be more boring than a grilled lamb chop, with its two teaspoonsful of meat content? Most meats are extremely boring to eat although, like other high-fat foods such as cheese, they do fill you up fast. The recipes in this book are not only highly nutritious, they are colourful and interesting as well. Many taste sensations in the diet are derived from eating foods that are interestingly spiced and lightly cooked. The recipes are low in salt, but do contain some. How much you add is really up to you, but they should not be oversalted like tinned soups and many prepared convenience dishes. In fact, after a few weeks on the anti-cellulite recipes, most bought processed foods will start to taste too salty.

Although there is no refined sugar in the recipes, a few contain raw sugar or organic honey. There is nothing wrong with eating these foods in extreme moderation, as in their unrefined state they contain some useful nutrients. You have to be careful, though, even with these, as there is addiction potential from all sugars. This is because they enter the bloodstream very quickly and deliver a drug-like 'high', which is then followed by a 'low', making you feel hungry and depressed.

The recipes in this book make you feel satisfied – and keep you satisfied for hours. It is not an exaggeration to say that you will feel a very different person if you make this your diet for life. The advantages of the diet include an end to severe mood swings, food-induced headaches and digestive problems. Not only will you look far better you will feel much happier and livelier as well.

This diet *must* be accompanied by large amounts of water – at least a litre a day, to rehydrate and detoxify the body. I can't emphasize this strongly enough. Since my original books were published, it has become clear that most of us are chronically dehydrated, and that this dehydration contributes to cellulite deposits being laid down – and staying there, because they cannot get out of the system, which has become sluggish like a pond full of weeds. Water moves rubbish as well as nutrients through the system, and we need to keep our own internal waterways clear and unclogged. The way to do this is to keep driving water through the system.

When people first start drinking more water, they often feel sick. This is because their bodies are having to get used to taking in more, and have become unaccustomed to it. If you feel sick when drinking extra water, don't gulp it down, but sip it. Also remember that if you fill a plastic bottle of water from the tap and leave it overnight in the fridge, the calcium will dissolve, and the water will taste almost indistinguishable from mineral water. We've almost come to believe that tap water is poisonous, but the problem is that if you always drink bought water, you may imagine you have no drinkable stuff when you run out.

Boiling water is just as effective as filtering it, and avoids the bother and expense of water filters.

A word about supplements: if your body is full of a lot of toxins, you may not be able to assimilate expensive vitamin and mineral supplements. Two that help here are B-complex and C, which both aid detoxification. Also, if you are losing weight quickly, take a good multi-vitamin daily to make up any loss of nutrients or weakness you might feel.

Chapter 12

How Long Will It Take?

The question everybody contemplating the anti-cellulite diet asks is: how long will it take to achieve results?

It would be wonderful if we could diet for one, or at the most two, days and then all the cellulite would be gone for ever. Unfortunately, it does not happen like that. For most people, cellulite deposits have built up gradually over the years and, having lodged themselves firmly in position, are most reluctant to disappear. That is why a dedicated and prolonged attack is necessary, and why you must establish a way of eating that will mean your cellulite does not stand a chance of coming back.

The length of time it will take you to rid your body of cellulite depends on many factors: how long the cellulite has been there, how dedicated you are to persisting with the diet as well as the other aspects – body brushing, aromatherapy and massage – and how much cellulite you have in the first place. No two people's metabolism is the same, and what works for one person will not necessarily have the same result in another.

For some very lucky people, cellulite disappears extremely quickly once they start the regime. In my case, it took a long time – about three months altogether. I didn't notice any real improvement until I had not only been on the diet, but also body-brushed rigorously and massaged with the correct aromatherapy oils for two months. However, once things began to happen, progress was rapid. Everybody noticed that there was something different about me, although of course they did not always know what it was.

For anyone who has had a cellulite problem for five years or more, two months is a reasonable length of time to wait before results become noticeable. For young women who have only just noticed puckers and dimples, a couple of weeks may make an appreciable difference.

It is most important to give your body a really good opportunity to yield up long-held cellulite, so you should stick to the cleansing diet for two weeks if you possibly can. This means no coffee or tea, no cream, cheese or other dairy products, no bread with gluten, no processed or prepared foods, nothing burnt, sautéed or fried, no frozen puddings, ice-cream, desserts, sugar, sweets, chocolate, alcohol or cigarettes.

This list seems endlessly long, but all the items above are definitely not cleansing ones – just the opposite in fact. You should, if you can manage it, have two or three days on fresh fruit alone. At the same time, drink as much mineral water as you can manage – eight glasses a day is not too much.

Fruit and vegetable juices are also good for you, but they need to be diluted and – it should go without saying – not sweetened in any way. Carrot and tomato juice, mixed vegetable juices, pineapple and apple juice will all help the cleansing process.

Don't forget that meat can be highly addictive food. It is one of the reasons it is so popular and people tend to feel deprived when they cannot have it. But meat is actually one of the easiest things to relinquish. Most people simply do not miss it after a while, so long as their meals are tasty, nutritious and filling without it. There is no harm in eating some meat, but you do not need it every day. Simple grilled or baked fish is an acceptable substitute.

The anti-cellulite diet has to be a diet for life. Otherwise, your cellulite will reappear and all your hard work will be wasted. Remember that cellulite is always trying to return and will take up residence again at the slightest provocation. Of course, there is no harm in the occasional indulgence in an ice-cream, a cream cake, or lasagne, but these should never again become part of your staple diet. If you have a propensity to cellulite then the diet is essential for you.

PART III
THE RECIPES

Chapter 13

Introduction to the Recipes

The best anti-cellulite diet is a strictly vegetarian one, where no animal products, including dairy products, are eaten at all. This is why I have devoted a special section to vegetarian meals. But apart from their general 'health-iness', vegetarian meals have several advantages over meat dishes. They are often quicker and easier to prepare and the ingredients are nicer to handle. They tend to be cheaper but, most important, *people enjoy them more!*

When I was first changing from being a carnivore to a vegetarian I often cooked two dishes, one non-meat and one containing meat, for dinner parties. I soon noticed that on every occasion the vegetarian dish dis-appeared within minutes and the meat dish was left. And my guests were by no means all vegetarian.

Vegetarian meals taste cleaner and lighter than meat ones, and are easier to digest. They don't leave a heavy feeling in the stomach, and many people find they have far more energy on a vegetarian diet.

However, for some people a sudden change to total vegetarianism is neither possible nor desirable. So I have included some anti-cellulite meat and fish dishes at the end of this section. They have been devised by Frances Clifford, the aromatherapist who helped me rid my thighs of the dread bulges and lumps, and who says she is nearly, but not quite, vegetarian herself. The more vegetarian meals you can introduce to your family the better it will be for them, as well as for you. If you do not want to eat meat or fish yourself but the rest of the family does, you can always cook lamb chops, chicken legs or sausages separately for them (or get some carnivore in the family to take responsibility for the meat ingredients).

The one golden rule on any anti-cellulite regime is: no high-fat dairy products. This means no eggs, double cream, full-cream milk, butter, or full-fat cheese. The only permissible dairy foods are low-fat yoghurt and quark, which can be eaten occasionally. You can even replace low-fat yoghurt with soya yoghurt, which in cooked food tastes exactly the same as the dairy variety. The reason for avoiding dairy products is that they are mucus-forming, which means they encourage cells and arteries to become clogged and blocked. Dairy products discourage quick through-put and elimination of food. Another factor is that these days many dairy foods are produced intensively, with the addition of hormones and chemicals, and these encourage the formation of cellulite.

Again, with several of the recipes other members of the family can add their own cheese or butter afterwards if they like.

The other important aspect of anti-cellulite cooking is that, as far as possible, you should not fry in oil or butter. This is in order to avoid the formation of free radicals.

Oils should preferably be monounsaturated, such as olive or rapeseed oil. Do not use artificially produced margarines if you can help it. A very small amount of butter does no harm, as long as you do not use it in cooking.

It is a culinary cliché that vegetables need to be sautéed first. However, this is done out of habit rather than necessity. For years I automatically stir-fried and sautéed everything, because this is what my vegetarian cookery books told me to do. When I started researching the recipes for this book I 'stir-fried' in water or stock instead, and found that the taste was just as good, if not better. The realization that vegetarian cookery does not need initial sautéeing was a revelation to me. When I served up dishes cooked in the new way, nobody noticed, and many were pronounced extra delicious.

Note: The quantities given in these recipes are for four people. But as this kind of cookery is not an exact science the quantities do not need to be followed exactly, especially with the vegetables. Spices are mainly a matter of taste, but err on the mean side at first, especially if the most exotic ingredients are new to you. In any case, anti-cellulite food should not be too highly spiced. Fresh herbs, which are now stocked by supermarkets should be bought in preference to dried, but as busy people do not always have time to shop for fresh herbs at every meal, quantities for dried equivalents are given as well, where appropriate.

Chapter 14

The Anti-Cellulite Kitchen

Not so very long ago, it would have been quite difficult to obtain the kind of store-cupboard items that are essential for an anti-cellulite kitchen. Now it is easy. The raw materials needed for this healthy way of cooking and eating are widely available from supermarkets and healthfood shops, and also, increasingly, from corner shops. The Indian revolution in corner shops has meant that so many previously exotic or difficult-to-obtain foods are now on sale in practically every town.

When establishing an anti-cellulite kitchen, the emphasis is on natural, additive-free, non-artificially coloured ingredients. Wherever possible, buy the real thing. Do not, for instance, buy instant coffee, but instead keep coffee beans in the freezer and grind them as you require them. It is now possible to buy decaffeinated beans, and also ready-ground decaffeinated filter coffee. The Nairobi Coffee Company produces a water-method decaffeinated filter coffee, in which the caffeine is flushed out of the beans with water. Instead of ordinary Indian tea, buy Luaka, in the mauve packet, which is real tea but low in tannin.

Get into the habit of buying herbal teas. There is now a huge variety available, so these drinks need never become boring.

All fruit and vegetable juices are good for you, so long as they do not contain added sugar. Always have a big bowl of fresh fruit and lots of fresh vegetables, preferably organically grown. All sprouted grains – alfalfa, mung, beansprouts etc – are good, but they go off very quickly indeed and should really be eaten the same day they are bought.

Buy soya or oat flour instead of wheat flour, and try carob powder instead of chocolate. Carob is rather like chocolate in taste, but is much lower in fat and sugar and is not addictive.

Your store cupboard should always contain seeds and unsalted nuts. Choose from sesame, pumpkin, poppy, caraway and sunflower seeds, pine kernels, almonds, brazils, cashews, chestnuts, walnuts, hazelnuts and pecans. Always buy fresh rather than salted nuts. Peanuts are not recommended on the anti-cellulite diet as they are acid-forming and heavy on the liver.

Keep on the look-out for bread and similar products that do not contain gluten. Rye bread, oatcakes, pumpernickel, barleycakes and puffed rice cakes are all good substitutes for bread.

Always buy brown rice rather than white and buckwheat spaghetti rather than the ordinary kind.

Barley can be used in all brown rice recipes for a change.

Do stock up on pulses. Lentils – red, green and brown – do not need soaking so they are worth buying in packets, but if you prefer you can buy tins of the other pulses – butter beans, chick peas, kidney beans etc – to save time. Generally I do not recommend tinned foods, but pulses other than lentils take ages to cook and seem to lose very little in the tinning process. Tins of chick peas and kidney beans are cheap and ready to use, and can be rinsed and added to any salad dish to make a satisfying meal.

Dairy products should be avoided as much as possible. Instead, get into the habit of buying soya milk and tofu – an unfermented soya-bean curd. Soya milk keeps for several months until opened, after which it must be treated like ordinary milk. Plamil and Granose are the big names to look out for in soya products. Granose also make a range of baby foods.

Don't forget Quorn, now available in pieces, mince and ready-made recipes. Quorn is low-fat mycoprotein, more versatile than meat, and can be used in all meat recipes. Just follow the instructions on the packet.

The only yogurt you should buy from now on is low-fat live plain yoghurt. This is very low in calories and also quite thick. Don't buy any cream – double, single, clotted or sour. Cow's milk should be skimmed or semi-skimmed. Plain cottage cheese, fromage frais, quark – a tasty soft cheese prepared with skimmed milk – and medium-fat vegetable rennet feta are the only acceptable cheeses from now on. Soya cheese, available from healthfood shops, is quite delicious and okay to use occasionally. Prewett's make a reduced-fat cheese, and you can obtain sunflower cheese as well.

Butter is better than margarine, simply because it's more natural and not highly processed. Always buy the unsalted kind, and use extremely sparingly. Do not use in cooking. The vegetable oils you use should be cold-pressed. Always use extra-virgin cold-pressed olive oil, sesame seed, grapeseed, sunflower or safflower oil. Olive oil has a strong taste, whereas sesame seed oil has hardly any taste at all, and so may be better in some recipes where the taste of olive oil is not really wanted.

There are no recipes in this book for eggs. I have not eaten eggs for ten years and have not missed them once. They are not necessary to your diet at all. But if you like them, it goes without saying that any you buy should be free-range, from hens that have been fed on organic produce.

Any meat, fish or poultry you buy should be from an organic source. You do not need meat or fish, but if you like it, or feel you cannot do without it, then eat it from time to time. Smoked meats, fish and cheese are OUT, because the smoking process results in free radicals.

Seasonings are of course extremely important in the anti-cellulite diet. Always buy sea salt and whole peppercorns. Keep a large supply of vegetable stock cubes or buy Vecon or Vegemite in jars. Fresh ginger root is used a lot in the recipes, as is garlic. I have discovered onion powder available from many supermarkets, for dips and patés, and it is wonderful. It does not contain any additives, and it saves having to be in floods of tears from chopping up onions all the time.

All the curry spices – turmeric, cumin, coriander, fenugreek, garam masala – are useful, especially when you are cooking low-salt recipes. Cinnamon, allspice, bay leaves, cloves, cayenne, dill, fennel, nutmeg, oregano, paprika, mustard seeds are all vital. Whenever possible, buy herbs such as basil, parsley, coriander, rosemary, sage and thyme fresh. Or grow them yourself, but keep the dried ones handy in case you run out – they're better than nothing.

All flavourings, such as vanilla essence, should be the real thing and not artificial substitutes. It is now becoming far easier to buy real essences. For a long time, only artificial versions were available – I can't imagine why.

Low-salt soya sauce is very handy as a flavouring. You can now also buy 'healthy' versions of tomato ketchup and Worcestershire sauce from healthfood shops.

Spreads and jams should not contain added sugar. I have grown to love sesame seed spread – tahini – and sunflower spread, which I now buy in preference to butter. Whole Earth jams and marmalades do not contain sugar but are quite sweet enough.

There are also now very many paste and pâtés available which are delicious and good for you. Look for olive paste, artichoke paste, and other vegetable pastes.

You will need a few gadgets, although these recipes do not require many at all: a coffee grinder is very useful for grinding up nuts as well as coffee beans, and a liquidizer is absolutely essential for many of the recipes. A fully fledged food processor is a good idea. Saucepans should not be made of aluminium. A steamer would be useful but is not essential. A garlic press is very useful too. An accurate pair of kitchen scales would help, but most of the recipes do not depend on absolutely accurate amounts.

There is no need whatever to count calories with these recipes. Although they are not all low-calorie, they will certainly discourage fat deposits from forming. They will leave you feeling pleasantly full and satisfied. It is not so easy to overeat brown rice as it is to gorge on pasta with cream sauces.

Convenience foods are not totally forbidden. I stock up on vegetarian sausages, quorn burgers, soya frankfurters, soya and mushroom burgers, and nut and sesame burgers. These are all made by Granose and are absolutely delicious. The Realeat company sells vegeburger mixes, soups and ready-made burgers. The instructions are for frying, but I heat them up in the microwave and they are just as nice, if not nicer. They are already cooked and, unlike meat burgers, it doesn't matter all that much if you do not heat them up.

If you have a freezer you can stock up on non-dairy ice-creams – I don't mean those made with whale oil or whatever, but soya frozen desserts. They taste almost the same as 'real' ice-cream, but without the fat content. Also it's a good idea to have frozen vegeburgers and sausages in the freezer for emergencies.

If you must each chocolate, go for Green and Black's Organic chocolate, or for one of the cheaper supermarket brands of chocolate containing 70 per cent (or thereabouts) cocoa. This is much less sweet than ordinary chocolate and a very small amount is satisfying.

Also, keep a lookout in your local health food shops for new, healthy spreads, pâtés, non-wheat pastas and rice noodles. The range is ever expanding. The kosher sections of supermarkets have wonderful humus, aubergine pâté, and so on. For some reason, the kosher versions seem to be tastier and nicer than other varieties. Organic pesto and other sauces for pasta are now available at most supermarkets.

Can't live your life without crisps? There are now crisps made from vegetables other than potatoes, which do not contain salt. Look out for them at your local health food shop or deli.

Brown rice used to take ages to prepare. However, you can now get Ready Rice – Whole Earth do a good range – and manufacturers such as Uncle Ben's have tins of ready-cooked brown rice. There is nothing wrong with these, and they save time.

Onion and garlic come ready-minced and in jars or tubes: there is nothing wrong with using these.

Over the past few year supermarkets have introduced ready-prepared salads. Marks and Spencer do a large range, as do Waitrose and Sainsbury's. These are very useful for those occasions when you do not have time to buy ingredients and chop them up. Most supermarkets now do very imaginative raw vegetable mixes, and although they may seem expensive they can work out cheaper than buying lots of salad ingredients you will only end up throwing away.

Most vegetables can be microwaved and, although some people are anti-microwave, I don't see anything wrong with them. Microwaving keeps all the flavour in, and also means you don't have to fry things.

All the recipes in this book are easy to prepare. There are no recipes for pastry, cakes, biscuits, bread, soufflés or roulades, for example. The emphasis is on dishes that are easy and quick to cook as well as appetizing and enjoyable to eat.

Chapter 15

Breakfast

It is often said that breakfast is the most important meal of the day and it is certainly the one I enjoy most. There is plenty of scope for the anti-cellulite breakfast to be both varied and delicious – and filling and satisfying at the same time.

Some people find they can start the day happily with a couple of bananas, and that these will keep them going throughout the morning. This sort of fare will not do at all for me, as I do not find it particularly filling. However, this is the time of day when you can eat a lot of fruit. Nathan Pritikin said that the liver likes fruit until lunch time, and this seems to have been confirmed by later researches. Eat most of your fruit in the morning; the later in the day you eat it, the harder your body finds it to digest.

If you are just starting the anti-cellulite regime, it is best to stick to one variety of fruit at a time rather than having a fruit cocktail, which can be hard work for the digestive system as all the fruits contain different substances. Although slimming diets commonly suggest starting the day with a grapefruit, most anti-cellulite experts do not recommend too much citrus fruit as the liver finds it quite hard to cope with. Grapefruit and oranges are very strong, and in addition contain large amounts of salicylic acid, the aspirin-like chemical that can lead to allergies. Most people find, however, that lemon juice does not cause these problems.

The fruit you eat can be as exotic as you like. Fruits such as papaya, guava, mango, pineapple, passion fruit, persimmon and melon are all wonderful at breakfast time. For a fairly substantial breakfast, grind up in a coffee grinder equal amounts of sunflower, pumpkin and sesame seeds and sprinkle these on the fruit. That will help to keep hunger pangs at bay for a little longer.

You can also keep whole sunflower and pumpkin seeds handy for snacks later during the day. It has been said that sunflower seeds help to reduce a craving for cigarettes, so if you are desperately trying to give up smoking, buy loads of sunflower seeds and have these instead.

Do try not to eat ordinary bread while on the strict anti-cellulite regime, and certainly don't have toast, butter and marmalade. Although for many people this is the standard British breakfast, it could not be worse from a cellulite point of view. First you have the bread, which contains gluten. This tends to clog up the intestines and can cause digestive problems. Then you compound the damage by toasting the bread, thus releasing free radicals. After that you spread on mucus-clogging butter and lastly, sugar-laden jam or marmalade. All in all, a highly processed and not very healthy start to the day.

It can be hard to persist with fruit and mineral water while everybody else is feasting on highly palatable breakfasts, but it will be worth it in the end. You will come to look forward to this light, energizing start to the day.

It is a good idea to get into the habit of not drinking at the same time as you are eating, as liquids tend to dilute the digestive juices, making it harder to digest food properly. When you first wake up, have a glass of mineral water or a wake-up herbal tea but do not drink with your breakfast.

You should not drink tea or coffee for the first two weeks of the anti-cellulite diet. Instead, have herbal tea or a coffee substitute. For a long time, I could not find any decent coffee substitutes, but now I have come across two that are really quite acceptable – Aromalt and Yannoh, both widely available from healthfood shops. No coffee substitute has quite the taste of the real thing, of course, but all serious cellulite-shifters must try to wean themselves off caffeine.

You can drink decaffeinated coffee so long as the caffeine has been removed by the water process – if it has, it will say so on the packet. Otherwise, you are just substituting one set of chemicals for other chemicals, which are probably just as harmful in their way.

Any cow's milk you buy should be skimmed or semi-skimmed. I now find that full-fat milk is too rich for me, and the skimmed variety is just right. So much of what we think we like is purely the result of ingrained habit, rather than absolute free choice.

If you possibly can, try to exist on fruit alone, or fruit plus ground natural seeds, for breakfast for a week. Then you can introduce more substantial fare, such as porridge, muesli and yoghurt-based shakes.

Porridge is a very good, healthy food for all the family, provided it is made in the traditional way, and not with lashings of milk, cream and sugar. You can add a small amount of organic honey, chopped dates or figs, or soaked Hunza apricots to the basic oat mixture. To make porridge, use twice the amount of water to porridge oats, bring to the boil then simmer, stirring all the time, until you have a smooth paste.

Muesli is also a good choice for breakfast, so long as it does not contain added sugar or any preservatives or additives. Many ready-made mueslis are very high in both fats and sugar, so read the label carefully first. Soak overnight in a little mineral water and then eat with live low-fat yoghurt in the morning.

One of my favourite breakfasts is a banana shake, quickly made in the liquidizer. All you do is empty the contents of a small carton of low-fat yoghurt (use soya yoghurt if you prefer) into the liquidizer, chop up a banana and add that, together with a squeeze of lemon juice and half a teaspoon of organic honey. Blend well until all is smooth, then serve topped with ground nuts. Or you could add a few dates, figs or soaked apricots.

You do not necessarily have to give up bread at the start of the day. Oatcakes, pumpernickel, rye and Manna bread (a sprouted, unleavened bread made without added salt, sugar or preservatives) are all acceptable gluten-free substitutes, or you can buy special gluten-free bread, which is now quite widely available. Oatcakes with sesame or sunflower seed spread will last just as long as hot buttered toast and marmalade, and once you have got used to them you may even find you prefer them. I do, now. Wholemeal pitta bread, which is unleavened, can be heated in the oven or microwave and then filled with sesame or sunflower spread.

If you must have jam or marmalade, try the Whole Earth varieties, which do not contain any sugar, although they are still high in calories.

Whatever you do, never go without breakfast. There is always the danger of snacking on junk food in the middle of the morning, and then making yourself feel horrible as a result. Breakfast need only take a very few minutes to prepare and eat, and it will set you up for hours. It is especially important to have a nutritious, non-cellulite-forming breakfast if you work in a place where you cannot easily get the right sort of food at lunch time. Staff canteens, school and college dining halls and sandwich bars are unlikely to be able to provide the kind of food you should ideally be eating. It is a good idea to take herbal tea bags and a coffee substitute into work, so that you do not succumb to the tealady's offerings.

Chapter 16

Soups

These soups are quick and easy to make. Unlike most recipes for soups, they do not rely on initial sautéeing in oil or butter. You may notice that they taste slightly different from the homemade soups you are used to, and the difference will be that they are lighter and fresher in taste.

The fresher the vegetables, the tastier the soups will be. These ones require little or no culinary skill, but most do need a food processor or liquidizer. Some people quite like soups with bits of vegetables swimming around in them – I prefer mine to be smooth.

Anyone just starting an anti-cellulite regime can safely eat all the soups here. If they are not quite filling enough you can always sprinkle on top a mixture of ground sunflower, sesame and pumpkin seeds. In fact, you should always keep a jar of this mixture handy to sprinkle over vegetables and soups, as it will stop you going for the bread and butter.

Chestnut Soup

This soup has a rather 'Christmassy' taste, but of course it can be eaten at any time of the year. It's very nutritious and filling, and extremely 'more-ish'.

6oz (175g) tinned or dried chestnuts – dried ones
will need soaking overnight
2 onions, chopped
2 carrots, finely chopped
2 sticks celery, chopped
½ teaspoon fresh thyme, or ¼ teaspoon dried
about ¼ nutmeg, grated
sea salt and freshly ground black pepper
1–1½ pints (600–900ml) vegetable stock (for tinned
chestnuts, otherwise use 2 pints (1.2l) water)
2 tablespoons chopped fresh parsley

PREPARATION TIME: 10 minutes
COOKING TIME: if using tinned chestnuts, about 45
minutes; otherwise 1½ hours. Note: with dried
chestnuts you have to think about this recipe 24
hours in advance.

If using dried chestnuts, put in a bowl and pour over 2 pints (1.2l) boiling water. Leave to soak for 24 hours, then put the chestnuts plus the soaking liquid in a large saucepan and add the onions, carrots and celery. Bring to the boil. If using tinned chestnuts, bring to the boil with the vegetable stock instead of water. Cover and simmer until tender – wait 1½ hours for dried chestnuts, 30 minutes for tinned. Allow to cool slightly, then liquidize. Return to the saucepan, and reheat gently with the thyme, nutmeg and seasoning. Do not allow to boil again. If the mixture is too thick, add more stock or water. Garnish with the parsley to serve.

Leek and Potato Soup

A quick, easy and satisfying soup for when leeks are in season.

> 1 medium onion, finely chopped
> 2 large leeks, washed and chopped
> 2 large potatoes, scrubbed and cubed
> 2oz (50g) ground cashews or hazelnuts
> 1 pint (600ml) vegetable stock
> pinch mixed dried herbs
> sea salt and freshly ground black pepper

PREPARATION TIME: 10 minutes
COOKING TIME: 35 minutes

Heat 2–3 tablespoons of the stock in a large saucepan. Add the onion, leeks, potatoes and nuts and stir-fry in the stock over a medium heat for 5 minutes. Bring to the boil and add the rest of the stock. Cover and simmer until the potatoes are cooked but still intact (about 25 minutes). Allow to cool slightly, then liquidize. Return to the saucepan and reheat gently with the herbs and seasoning. Do not boil.

Watercress Soup

Watercress gives a pungent taste to this satisfying soup.

1½ pints (900ml) vegetable stock
1 large onion, finely chopped
1 clove garlic, crushed
1lb (450g) potatoes, scrubbed and cubed
large pinch mixed dried herbs
sea salt and freshly ground black pepper
1 bunch watercress, washed and chopped

PREPARATION TIME: 10 minutes
COOKING TIME: 35 minutes

Heat 3–4 tablespoons of the vegetable stock in a large saucepan then add the onion, garlic and potatoes. Cook on a medium heat for 5 minutes, then bring to the boil. Add the herbs, salt and pepper, and cook until the potatoes are tender – about 20 minutes. Add the watercress and cook for a further 5 minutes. Cool slightly, then liquidize. Return to the saucepan and reheat gently, stirring in more stock or water if the soup is too thick.

Carrot Soup

Another 'main meal' soup, colourful, filling and tasty.

    1 large onion, chopped
    1 clove garlic, crushed
    1 sprig fresh rosemary, chopped, or ¼ teaspoon
    dried rosemary
    1lb (450g) carrots, finely chopped
    1½ pints (900ml) vegetable stock
    ¼ teaspoon mild curry powder
    1 tablespoon medium oatmeal
    sea salt

PREPARATION TIME: 5 minutes
COOKING TIME: 30 minutes

Cook the onion, garlic, rosemary and carrots in 2–3 tablespoons stock over a medium heat for about 5 minutes, then bring to the boil. Add the rest of the stock, the curry powder, oatmeal and salt, then cover the saucepan, lower the heat, and simmer for about 20 minutes or until the carrots are soft. Blend in a liquidizer then return to the saucepan, reheating gently. Add more stock or water if the soup is too thick.

Brussels Sprout Soup with Yoghurt

If you like Brussels sprouts, you'll love this soup.

1¼ pints (900ml) vegetable stock
1lb (450g) Brussels sprouts, trimmed and finely chopped
1 large onion, finely chopped
sea salt and freshly ground black pepper
2 strips lemon rind
2 teaspoons soya flour
1 carton low-fat natural live yoghurt or plain soya yoghurt
3 tablespoons chopped fresh parsley

PREPARATION TIME: 10 minutes
COOKING TIME: 35 minutes

Heat 2–3 tablespoons of the stock in a large saucepan and sweat the sprouts and onions over a medium heat, stirring all the time, for 10 minutes. Add the remaining stock and bring to the boil. Lower the heat, season, add the lemon rind, then cover and simmer for about 20 minutes. Remove the lemon rind, liquidize the soup then return to the saucepan. Mix the soya flour with the yoghurt then stir into the soup with the parsley. Do not allow to boil, or the yoghurt may curdle.

Jerusalem Artichoke Soup

Jerusalem artichokes are knobbly and offputting in appearance, but make delightful soups. Here is a very simple recipe.

1 pint (600ml) vegetable stock
2–3 large leeks, washed and chopped
1lb (450g) artichokes, scrubbed or peeled, and chopped
2 medium carrots, diced
1 bay leaf
1 teaspoon fresh or ½ teaspoon dried basil
1 clove garlic, crushed
sea salt and freshly ground black pepper

PREPARATION TIME: 10 minutes
COOKING TIME: 25 minutes

Put the stock in a saucepan with the vegetables and bring to the boil. Add the herbs, garlic and seasoning, lower the heat and simmer for about 20 minutes, or until the artichokes are cooked. Liquidize, then return to the saucepan and reheat gently. Do not boil as this impairs the flavour.

Spinach and Tofu Soup

A light and creamy soup which requires minimal cooking time.

2¼ pints (1.35l) vegetable stock
2 packs Tofeata or Morinaga tofu, drained and cut
into cubes
2lb (900g) spinach, washed and roughly chopped
sea salt and freshly ground black pepper
chopped fresh parsley to garnish

PREPARATION TIME: 5 minutes
COOKING TIME: 20 minutes

Bring the stock to the boil in a pan. Add the tofu and spinach and bring back to the boil, then cover and simmer for 10 minutes, stirring occasionally. Liquidize if liked, when cooled slightly. Add salt and pepper and reheat. Sprinkle the chopped parsley over the soup just before serving.

Green Split Pea Soup

Versatile split peas, available very cheaply from any supermarket, can easily be made into appetizing soups.

12oz (350g) dried green split peas
½ green pepper, chopped
1½ pints (900ml) vegetable stock
1 stick celery, finely chopped
1 medium onion, chopped
1 carrot, finely chopped or grated
½ teaspoon fresh or ¼ teaspoon dried marjoram
sea salt and freshly ground black pepper

PREPARATION TIME: 10–15 minutes
COOKING TIME: about 2¼ hours (but you don't have
to stand over it all the time)

In a large saucepan, bring the split peas and green pepper to the boil in the stock. Lower the heat and simmer very gently for about 1¼ hours. Add the remaining ingredients and simmer for another 45 minutes, or until everything is tender. Liquidize if liked, after cooling slightly, then reheat and check the seasoning.

Chapter 17

Starters and Dips

Although classed as starters, many of these dishes make complete light meals in themselves. They are particularly suitable for lunches, for when you are on your own, or when you haven't much time to prepare a full-scale meal. Although they are all anti-cellulite not all these dishes are low-calorie.

When recipes specify olive oil make sure you always use one labelled 'extra-virgin'. It is slightly more expensive but it really is worth it. Although olive oil is the best sort of oil to use, as it is monounsaturated, it does have rather a strong taste and if you don't like it you can substitute a cold-pressed sesame or grapeseed oil, which have hardly any taste at all.

Hummous

There are many versions of hummous, a Greek dish based on chick peas. Over the years I must have tried them all, and this one is my favourite.

1 14oz (400g) tin chick peas, drained and rinsed (or
you can cook your own according to the instructions on page 280)
1 dessertspoon tahini
juice 1 lemon
1 clove garlic, crushed
2 tablespoons olive oil
1 tablespoon low-fat natural yoghurt
1 dessertspoon chopped fresh parsley
sea salt and freshly ground black pepper
paprika to garnish

PREPARATION TIME: about 5 minutes
COOKING TIME: nil

This must be one of the easiest dishes ever devised, if
you have a liquidizer. If not, I should imagine it's mur-
der. Simply put all the ingredients except the paprika
into the liquidizer and blend on top speed until a
smooth paste is formed. Turn into a suitable dish and
garnish with paprika.

Serve with crudités – sticks of carrot and celery,
chunks of broccoli or cauliflower, and green and red
peppers. You can also serve hummous with manna or
gluten-free bread, or spread on oatcakes or barleycakes. You will not need to spread butter or margarine
on first.

Avocado Dip

Avocados are high in fat, but they do not encourage cellulite to form. This dip is good with crudités, or it can be spread on manna bread or oatcakes, like the hummous.

1 large ripe avocado
1 pack tofu
juice of 1 lemon, or to taste
2 tablespoons cold-pressed sunflower or grapeseed oil
sea salt and freshly ground black pepper

PREPARATION TIME: about 5 minutes
COOKING TIME: nil

Peel and stone the avocado and chop into small pieces. Break up the tofu in a bowl. Put all the ingredients in a blender and blend until smooth. Serve with raw carrots, broccoli, etc, as for hummous.

Sunflower Dip

4oz (125g) sunflower seeds, ground
1 clove garlic, crushed
1 stick celery, very finely chopped
juice ½ lemon

PREPARATION TIME: 5 minutes
COOKING TIME: nil

Blend all the ingredients in a liquidizer on high speed.
Add spring water to make this dip more runny if necessary.

Cashew and Tofu Pâté

This is a more 'festive', sophisticated pâté, for special
occasions or dinner parties.

2 tablespoons vegetable stock
1 small onion or shallot, very finely chopped
1 clove garlic, crushed
1 pack Morinaga or Tofeata tofu
4oz (125g) ground cashew nuts
1 tablespoon olive oil
4 tablespoons spring or filtered water (or, for a very
special occasion, you could use white wine)
2 tablespoons chopped fresh parsley, or (in an
emergency) 2 teaspoons dried
sea salt and freshly ground black pepper

PREPARATION TIME: about 10 minutes
COOKING TIME: 5 minutes

Heat the vegetable stock in a saucepan and gently stir-fry the onion and garlic over a medium heat until softened. Remove from the heat. In a large mixing bowl, mash the tofu with a fork, then add the onion and garlic. Now add the nuts, olive oil, water or wine, parsley, salt and pepper and stir well. Press the pâté into 1 large or 4 small earthenware dishes and chill in the fridge for an hour or two, if possible, before serving.

Quark and Walnut Dip

Although the emphasis of this book is on non-dairy foods, quark – the low-fat cheese made with skimmed milk – does no harm occasionally. This dip tastes much creamier and more calorific than it actually is. The onions are essential.

8oz (225g) quark
1 tablespoon olive oil
sea salt and freshly ground black pepper
1 small onion, very finely chopped, or 1 teaspoon onion granules
1 tablespoon chopped fresh parsley
2oz (50g) walnuts, ground

PREPARATION TIME: 10 minutes
COOKING TIME: nil

Put all the ingredients into a liquidizer and blend on high speed until completely homogenized. If the dip is too thick, add a little spring water or skimmed milk and blend again.

Aubergine and Tahini Dip

Although aubergines taste wonderful in dips, they are rather a nuisance to prepare, as they take ages. However, once in a while it is worth taking the trouble to make this delicious dip.

1 large or 2 small aubergines
2 tablespoons tahini
juice 1 lemon
1 clove garlic, crushed
2 tablespoons finely chopped fresh parsley
sea salt and freshly ground black pepper

PREPARATION TIME: 10 minutes
COOKING TIME: 1 hour

Preheat the oven to 350°F, 180°C, gas mark 4. Bake the aubergine for about 1 hour, or until soft – test with a fork. Hold the aubergine under the cold tap and peel off the purple skin. Then put all the ingredients into a liquidizer and blend on high speed. Transfer to a glass or earthenware container and chill for an hour or two,

if possible, although the dip can be eaten straight away
if required.

Vegetable Pâté

This pâté can be eaten by itself, with a salad, used as a
dip or as a spread on oatmeal biscuits.

1 stick celery, chopped
½ cucumber, chopped
1 medium green pepper, chopped
1 medium onion, finely chopped
½ teaspoon fresh or dried dill weed
4oz (125g) cottage cheese or quark
sea salt and freshly ground black pepper

PREPARATION TIME: 5 minutes
COOKING TIME: nil

Place all the ingredients in a liquidizer and blend on
high speed until a smooth paste is formed – it won't be
completely smooth, though.

Asparagus with Yoghurt Dressing

This is a healthy version of the more usual asparagus
with melted butter or hollandaise sauce.

1 small onion, finely chopped, or ½ teaspoon onion
powder
½ clove garlic, crushed
juice ½ lemon
1 carton low-fat live yoghurt
1 large bunch asparagus

PREPARATION TIME: 5 minutes
COOKING TIME: about 10 minutes

First, make the yoghurt dressing by mixing together
the onion, garlic, lemon juice and yoghurt. Then trim
the asparagus and boil in salted water until tender –
about 10 minutes. Drain, and serve warm with the
yoghurt dressing.

Quick and Easy Burgers

These burgers do not need cooking and, with a salad,
make a complete meal in themselves.

4oz (125g) cashews, almonds or mixed nuts, ground
8oz (225g) quark or cottage cheese
3 tablespoons chopped fresh parsley
1 small onion, grated or finely chopped – or use ¼
teaspoon onion granules
sea salt and freshly ground black pepper
wholemeal breadcrumbs for coating

PREPARATION TIME: about 5 minutes
COOKING TIME: nil

In a large mixing bowl combine the ground nuts,
quark or cottage cheese, parsley, onion and seasoning.
The mixture will be fairly stiff. Divide into 4 and form
into burger shapes. Roll in breadcrumbs and put in the
fridge until required.

Raita

This version of the well-known cool accompaniment to
hot Indian dishes is also good as a dip in its own right.

½ cucumber, finely chopped
sea salt and freshly ground black pepper
1 teaspoon caraway seeds
1 tablespoon fresh mint, chopped
2–3 spring onions, finely chopped
1 carton low-fat live yoghurt

PREPARATION TIME: 5 minutes
COOKING TIME: nil

Mix all the ingredients together well and serve immediately.

Mushrooms à la Grecque

A sophisticated starter – but you've got to like garlic.

¼ pint (150ml) water
2 cloves garlic, crushed
juice 2 lemons
2 tablespoons olive oil
1 bay leaf
sea salt and freshly ground black pepper
12oz (350g) button mushrooms
1 firm tomato, skinned and chopped
2 tablespoons chopped fresh parsley

PREPARATION TIME: 10 minutes
COOKING TIME 10 minutes

Put all the ingredients except the parsley, mushrooms and tomato into a saucepan, bring to the boil and boil for 5 minutes. Add the mushrooms, lower the heat and simmer for another 5 minutes. Remove from the heat and add the chopped tomato. Sprinkle with the parsley. Allow to cool, then refrigerate for an hour or two before serving.

Stuffed Tomatoes

Shirley Conran is famous for saying that life is too short to stuff a mushroom. But it's not too short to stuff a tomato, and this delicious recipe takes hardly any time at all. Tomatoes can also be stuffed with rice salad (see pages 245–246).

4 large, firm tomatoes (don't choose really huge ones, but they must be firm)
4oz (125g) wholemeal breadcrumbs
4oz (125g) quark, cottage or other low-fat soft cheese, such as fromage frais
2 tablespoons finely chopped chives
sea salt and freshly ground black pepper
parsley to garnish

PREPARATION TIME: 7–8 minutes
COOKING TIME: nil

Cut a lid off the top of the tomatoes and carefully scoop out the flesh, making sure you don't cut the outside of the tomatoes. Chop the pulp and transfer to a mixing bowl. Add all the remaining ingredients except the parsley and mix well. Fill the tomatoes with the mixture, garnish with parsley, and replace the lids. Serve chilled.

Chapter 18

Salads and Dressings

Salads are, of course, the mainstay of the anti-cellulite diet. Even if you haven't always got the time or the ingredients for a full-scale salad, you should make sure you have something raw at every meal, as to some extent this will work to detoxify any less healthy food you might have eaten or be about to eat.

However, in the anti-cellulite diet salads are the stars, rather than being relegated to bit-players. The whole concept of what constitutes a salad has undergone a dramatic change in recent years, and these days they can be complete and satisfying meals in themselves.

When possible, make sure the salad ingredients are really fresh and organically grown. Organic produce tastes quite different from the other kind, even if its appearance may not be quite so attractive.

It is important that salads should be colourful, as this makes them look more appetizing. Fortunately this is easy, as the raw ingredients tend to be colourful in their own right. Always make sure your salad has a variety of colours.

Do get into the habit of buying fresh sprouted grains, such as beansprouts, alfalfa or others, now available from most supermarkets. You can even sprout your own, and many vegetarian cookery books have instructions for doing this. I have found that the bought sprouts are just as good as the ones you attempt yourself. Sprouted grains can be strewn over the top of just about any salad – you don't need special recipes on how to use them. However, they don't last very long and should be eaten either on the day of purchase or the next day.

Sprouted grains contain many important nutrients, and all have a slight pea/beany taste, so they won't seem as unfamiliar as all that. Otherwise, look carefully at the salad section in your supermarket or greengrocer's. You will find that there is far more available these days than limp lettuce, tomatoes and cucumber. There are now many different types of salad greens around, and these all add interest and taste to a salad.

Once you have got into the habit of eating a salad at every meal you will soon find that you miss it if it is not there. Salad ingredients are not expensive, and even the most pricy lettuce or exotic vegetables will be far cheaper than junk foods and processed meats.

Here are some ideas for salads, and also for unusual dressings to accompany them. There is no need to peel the vegetables unless specifically instructed to do so by the recipe. Do avoid bought mayonnaise and salad dressings; they contain huge amounts of fat, and probably artificial preservatives as well.

Preparation times are not given in this section, as the salads take only minutes to prepare.

Nut and Rice Salad

8oz (225g) brown rice, cooked
4oz (125g) red cabbage, grated
1 green pepper, finely chopped
1 carrot, grated
1oz (25g) chopped nuts – hazels, almonds
or cashews
1oz (25g) sultanas

Mix all the ingredients together and serve with one of the dressings on pages 255–260.

Kidney Bean and Rice Salad

This is an extremely healthy and filling salad, containing lots of soluble fibre in the form of fresh vegetables and brown rice, all mixed together in a harmonious whole.

1 tin red kidney beans, drained – any size will do
4oz (125g) cooked brown rice

½ iceberg lettuce, washed and sliced or torn into
strips
2 sticks celery, very finely chopped
½ cucumber, washed and very finely chopped
vinaigrette (see page 255)

Combine all the ingredients together, mixing well and
adding just enough vinaigrette to coat the ingredients,
but not so there is dressing swimming at the bottom.
Note: you could use other pulses for this salad, such as
chick peas or butter beans, but kidney beans are the
most flavourful, as well as the most colourful. You can
spoon this salad into hot pitta bread if you like.

Walnut Salad with Figs

A very satisfying salad, and it's even nicer with fresh
figs than with dried.

¼ small white cabbage, grated
4 carrots, grated
1 onion, very finely chopped
1 cooking apple, grated
yoghurt or tofu dressing (see pages 257, 260)
4oz (125g) fresh or dried figs, sliced
2 dessert apples, finely sliced
juice 1 orange
4oz (125g) walnut pieces

Mix together the cabbage, carrots, onion and cooking apple. Stir in the dressing, mix well together, then arrange the slices of figs and dessert apples on top. Pour over the orange juice then scatter the walnuts over the salad.

Waldorf Salad

This salad is a universal favourite.

　　2 large dessert apples, cored and sliced
　　2 sticks celery, washed and sliced
　　2oz (50g) walnuts
　　2oz (50g) hazelnuts
　　2oz (50g) sultanas
　　chopped fresh parsley
　　yoghurt dressing (see page 260)

Mix the apples, celery, nuts, sultanas and parsley together and combine with the yoghurt dressing.

Date Salad

A wonderfully colourful and tasty salad which will cheer you up if you need cheering up.

½ iceberg lettuce, washed and sliced or torn into
strips
4 oranges, peeled and thinly sliced
4oz (125g) dates, stoned and finely chopped. Use
fresh ones if possible – they are getting more widely
available all the time
2oz (50g) flaked almonds
lemon dressing (see page 255)

Put the lettuce in a serving bowl and arrange the
orange slices, dates and almonds on top. Pour the
lemon dressing over, but not so much that it swims at
the bottom.

New Potato Salad

An exciting way to use new potatoes when they first
come into season.

1lb (450g) new potatoes
2 tablespoons chopped fresh mint
tofu dressing (see page 257)

Cook the potatoes in boiling salted water until tender,
then rinse under the tap in a colander to cool. Cut into
small pieces and mix in a bowl with the mint and the
tofu dressing. Keep in the fridge until required, then
serve with a green salad.

Carrot Salad with Apples

juice ½ lemon
3 dessert apples, cored and sliced
1lb (450g) carrots, grated
3 tablespoons raisins
1 tablespoon sunflower seeds
2 tablespoons broken cashew nuts
½ iceberg lettuce, washed and sliced or torn into strips
vinaigrette (see page 255)

Sprinkle the lemon juice over the apples to prevent discoloration then mix with the carrots, raisins, sunflower seeds and nuts. Put the lettuce in a bowl, add the carrot, nut and apple mixture, then toss in the vinaigrette dressing.

Mixed Salad

Green salads can consist of just lettuce, cucumber and green peppers. This salad is slightly more special.

½ iceberg lettuce, washed and sliced or torn into strips
1 bunch watercress, washed and chopped
2–3 spring onions, finely chopped
2 courgettes, grated

2 carrots, grated
4 tomatoes, sliced
sunflower or pumpkin seeds
sunflower, vinaigrette, tofu or tahini dressing
(see pages 255, 256, 257)

Combine all the salad ingredients and toss in the vinaigrette, tofu or tahini dressing.

Experiment with other green leaves in salads – the choice has never been wider. Choose from lamb's lettuce, cos lettuce, Chinese leaves, radicchio – a strong, red lettuce which has made its appearance in British supermarkets recently – chicory, spinach leaves (use raw), nasturtium leaves, celery leaves, dandelion leaves (as long as they are young and very green). It is a good idea to keep a wooden bowl specially for green salads. Rub a clove of garlic round the inside first, and then just wipe after using. It should not need washing up.

Other vegetables can easily be added to a green salad – raw cauliflower or broccoli florets, or avocado slices, for example. Nuts, such as walnuts or hazelnuts, can also be added.

Greek Salad

You can now buy low-fat vegetarian feta cheese, which makes this popular Greek salad suitable for cellulite-shifters. Don't buy the high-fat, animal-rennet variety.

1 pack vegetarian feta cheese
½ iceberg lettuce, washed and sliced or torn into
strips
½ cucumber, cut into chunks
4–5 firm tomatoes, cut into chunks
12 black olives
vinaigrette dressing (see page 255)

In a glass bowl, combine all the salad ingredients and
toss in the vinaigrette dressing.

Pine Nut Salad

Once a rare delicacy, pine nuts are now easily available, and have a rich, rather slippery, taste when fresh.

4 tomatoes, chopped
6 radishes, finely chopped
½ iceberg lettuce, washed and sliced or torn into
strips
3 tablespoons finely chopped fresh parsley
1 packet alfalfa sprouts
3oz (75g) pine nuts
vinaigrette or yoghurt dressing (see pages 255, 260)

Mix all the salad ingredients together and toss in vinaigrette or yoghurt dressing.

Leek and Hazelnut Salad

Leeks are one of my favourite vegetables. They need a very little cooking for this salad, but not much, and certainly not enough to affect the vitamin content.

2 large leeks, washed and sliced in rings
1 red pepper, seeded and sliced
2oz (50g) hazelnuts, chopped
sea salt and freshly ground black pepper
vinaigrette or yoghurt dressing (see pages 255, 260)

Blanch the leeks in boiling salted water for 2 minutes, then cool by rinsing under the cold tap in a colander. Arrange the leeks, pepper and hazelnuts in a glass bowl, season, and toss in vinaigrette or yoghurt dressing.

Coleslaw

There are many ways of making coleslaw, but this one is tasty as well as healthy.

½ white cabbage, grated or finely sliced
2 large carrots, grated
½ teaspoon caraway seeds
freshly ground black pepper
yoghurt or tofu dressing (see pages 257, 260)

Combine all the ingredients, including the dressing, in a bowl. This coleslaw will keep for up to 4 days in the fridge, if kept covered.

Cauliflower Salad

Cauliflower can be eaten raw – as crudités, for example – but if preferred, can be steamed for about 5 minutes first for this salad. The dates give a 'comforting' feel to this vegetable and fruit combination.

    1 small or ½ large cauliflower, cut into small florets
    2oz (50g) dates, either dried or fresh
    2 bananas, sliced
    1 packet alfalfa sprouts
    tofu, yoghurt or tahini dressing (see pages 257, 258, 260) or
    soya mayonnaise (see page 259)

If steaming the cauliflower first, cook for 5 minutes then cool quickly by rinsing in a colander under the cold tap. Combine all the salad ingredients in a mixing bowl then add the dressing of your choice (they all go well).

Raw Beetroot Salad

8oz (225g) raw beetroot, peeled and grated
2 sticks celery, very finely chopped
2 large dessert apples, cored and chopped
vinaigrette or tahini dressing (see pages 255, 258)

Combine the beetroot, celery and apples then mix in
the dressing – just enough to moisten the salad.

Spinach and Cauliflower Salad

This salad uses raw cauliflower, so make sure all the
florets are very crisp and crunchy, and don't leave in
any woody cauliflower stems.

8oz (225g) new potatoes, cooked with mint, then
cooled
1 medium cauliflower, cut into very small florets
1lb (450g) spinach, washed and torn into strips
2–3 dessert apples, cored and sliced
2oz (50g) sunflower or soya cheese, cubed or sliced
vinaigrette dressing (see below)

If the potatoes are very tiny, leave whole. Otherwise,
slice them and mix with the remaining salad ingredients. Toss in the vinaigrette.

DRESSINGS

Vinaigrette Dressing

It is a good idea to make up this dressing in advance and then keep it in a screwtop jar in the fridge until required. It keeps well, and is suitable for most salads.

6 fl oz (175ml) cold-pressed olive oil, or other cold-pressed oil
3 fl oz (75ml) white wine vinegar
½ teaspoon honey
½ teaspoon sea salt
½ teaspoon freshly ground black pepper
1 teaspoon fresh or ½ teaspoon dried tarragon
½ teaspoon made mustard

Put all the ingredients in a bottle with a screwtop lid and shake thoroughly. This dressing is best left a day or two before use for the flavours to meld together. Before using, shake thoroughly again.

Lemon Dressing

juice 1 lemon
twice as much cold-pressed olive, safflower or sunflower seed oil as lemon juice
a little sea salt and freshly ground black pepper

Mix all the ingredients together. This dressing is good if you are just starting an anti-cellulite regime. You can even just squeeze the juice of a lemon on a salad if you like.

Avocado and Cashew Dressing

4oz (125g) cashew nuts, ground
½ avocado
juice ½ lemon
sea salt and freshly ground black pepper
½ onion, very finely chopped or grated
¼ pint (150ml) water

Blend all the ingredients in a liquidizer. Add only a very small amount of water at first, then keep adding as required, while the liquidizer is on high speed, until the desired consistency is reached. This dressing is very rich, and a little goes a long way.

Sunflower Seed Dressing

A lighter dressing which goes very well with green salads.

4oz (125g) sunflower seeds, ground
1 clove garlic, crushed

1 stick celery, very finely chopped
juice ½ lemon
water

Blend all the ingredients in a liquidizer, adding water slowly until the required consistency is obtained.

Tofu Dressing

This dressing looks exactly like mayonnaise, and can be used in all salad recipes where mayonnaise is specified.

1 pack tofu, drained
1 tablespoon cold-pressed olive oil
1 teaspoon lemon juice
1 tablespoon very finely chopped onion, or use onion powder
1 teaspoon honey
sea salt and freshly ground black pepper to taste

Put all the ingredients in a liquidizer and blend until smooth.

Tahini Dressing

Tahini, available from healthfood shops, is sesame seed paste and is very useful in an anti-cellulite diet. Over the years it has become indispensable to me and I've grown to love it. It tastes something like peanut butter but has more of an edge to it.

¼ pint (150ml) tahini
1 carton natural low-fat or soya yoghurt
juice 1 lemon
1 clove garlic, crushed, or use onion powder
2–3 tablespoons chopped fresh parsley
¼ teaspoon cayenne pepper
sea salt to taste

Liquidize all the ingredients together on high speed until smooth. This dressing will keep for up to three days in the fridge.

Cashew Dressing

4oz (125g) cashew nuts, ground
1 cup filtered water
2 cloves garlic, crushed, or use onion powder
juice 1 lemon
1 teaspoon Vecon

Blend all the ingredients together in a liquidizer on high speed. This dressing is a good substitute for mayonnaise.

Soya Mayonnaise

Beware with this one – it's horribly delicious. I first came across it in The Country Life restaurant in Heddon Street, London W1, which is run by the vegan Seventh-Day Adventists. The only way I can stop myself pigging on this mayonnaise is to make only very minute quantities. However, for four people you will need:

  1 carton soya milk
  1 teaspoon sea salt
  1 teaspoon onion powder or finely chopped onion
  8 fl oz (250ml) olive oil
  2 tablespoons lemon juice
  1–2 tablespoons chopped fresh parsley, or use
  oregano, basil or thyme

Blend the soya milk, salt and onion on high speed. As the blender is whirring round, pour in the olive oil very slowly. The more oil you pour, the thicker the mayonnaise will become. Transfer to a mixing bowl and fold the lemon juice and herbs into the mixture. This can be used like ordinary mayonnaise on salads, in jacket potatoes, or as a spread on wholemeal bread. It keeps for three or four days in a screwtop jar in the fridge.

Yoghurt Dressing

1 carton low-fat yoghurt
1 onion, finely chopped, or 1 teaspoon onion granules
½ clove garlic, crushed
juice ½ lemon
sea salt and freshly ground black pepper

Mix all the ingredients together or blend in a liquidizer.

Simple Avocado Dressing

½ large avocado, or 1 whole small one, peeled and stoned
juice ½ lemon
1 clove garlic, crushed
¼ teaspoon onion powder
sea salt and freshly ground black pepper

Blend all the ingredients together in a liquidizer. If the mixture is too stiff, add water rather than more lemon juice.

Chapter 19

Vegetarian Main Courses

JACKET POTATOES

These are the easiest vegetables to start you off on an anti-cellulite cookery regime. Try to buy organically grown potatoes if possible – as with other vegetables, this is getting easier all the time.

Cooking potatoes in their jackets conserves all their goodness – especially as most of the nutrients are found in or near the skin – and it is simplicity itself. Just preheat the oven to 400°F, 200°C, or gas mark 6, scrub the potatoes, prick with a fork and cook at the top of the oven for about an hour. Do not rub with butter or cover in aluminium foil (which is now being associated with the degeneration of tissues). If you use a microwave, jacket potatoes will take about 10 minutes to cook, according to size.

Cellulite-shifters should eat their potatoes with a salad, or one of the dips in the chapter on Starters and Dips. The rest of the family can add all the butter and cheese they like. Jacket potatoes can accompany any dish at all, and are a wonderful standby. They also leave everybody feeling pleasantly full, and I have yet to come across somebody who doesn't like them.

Cellulite-shifters should not ever eat chips or mash their potatoes with cream, milk or butter. You can mash them with a little low-fat yoghurt if you like, but that's all.

CURRIES

Curries are extremely easy to prepare and have the advantage of making ordinary vegetables tastier and more special. Many vegetables become easier to eat when delicately spiced, but don't overdo the spices in the belief that the more you add, the more exotic the dish will taste. The idea is to complement the natural taste of the vegetables. Once you've cooked a few of the curries suggested below, you will soon notice a difference between the home-cooked variety and those traditionally served in Indian restaurants, which tend to be oily and highly salted. *Always* use brown rice. It takes a little longer to cook than white, although many of the newer types of brown rice on sale are 'quick-cook', but the difference in taste is worth it. Once you are used to brown rice you will never want to go back to the white variety again.

Carrot and Mushroom Curry

This curry is delicately spiced and the spices complement, rather than overpower, the taste of the vegetables.

8oz (225g) brown rice
4 cups water (double the quantity of rice)
1 level teaspoon sea salt, or to taste
½ pint (300ml) vegetable stock, either homemade or made with Vecon or other vegetable concentrate
1 teaspoon grated or finely chopped fresh ginger root, or ¼ teaspoon powdered ginger
1 teaspoon ground turmeric
1 teaspoon ground cumin
1 teaspoon ground coriander
2 medium onions, finely chopped
2 large tomatoes, skinned
4 large carrots, finely chopped
8oz (225g) mushrooms, chopped – use large, flat, open mushrooms, if possible
1 teaspoon garam masala
sea salt to taste
2 tablespoons chopped coriander leaves to garnish (optional – but recommended)

PREPARATION TIME: about 15 minutes
COOKING TIME: 25–30 minutes altogether, depending on type of brown rice used. Holland and Barrett sell excellent quick-cooking brown rice.

Put the rice, cold water and sea salt in a pan and bring to the boil, lower the heat and simmer until tender. Meanwhile prepare the vegetables: pour half the stock into a large saucepan on a medium heat. Add the ginger, turmeric, cumin, coriander and onions, stirring all the time. Cook for about 10 minutes, then add the rest of the stock and the tomatoes, carrots and mushrooms. Bring to the boil, then lower the heat and simmer for about 25 minutes or until the vegetables are cooked. Stir in the garam masala, add salt and continue to cook for another minute. Stir in the coriander leaves if used and serve straight away with the rice.

This curry should be served with a salad. Low-fat yoghurt or raita (see page 240) can also be served as an accompaniment.

Broccoli, Sesame Seed and Brown Rice Curry

A quick, easy and tasty favourite.

½ pint (300ml) vegetable stock, made with Vecon or vegetable stock cube
1lb (450g) broccoli, chopped
8oz (225g) mushrooms, washed and chopped
2 tablespoons sesame seeds
sea salt and freshly ground black pepper
1 level teaspoon mild curry powder or garam masala
8oz (225g) brown rice, cooked

PREPARATION TIME: about 10 minutes
COOKING TIME: about 20 minutes

Heat about ¼ pint (150ml) of the stock in a saucepan and add the broccoli. Stir-fry for 3 minutes, then add the chopped mushrooms and stir for another 2 minutes. Add the remaining stock, bring to the boil then cover and simmer until the broccoli is just tender – about 10 minutes. Add the sesame seeds, salt and pepper and stir for 1 minute. Add the rice and curry powder and stir until thoroughly heated through. Serve at once with a mixed salad.

Note: the rice for this dish is even nicer if cooked in vegetable stock rather than plain water.

Spinach Curry

As you proceed with the anti-cellulite regime you will probably find yourself buying lots and lots of spinach. Fresh is best, of course, but frozen leaf spinach comes a very close second. Don't forget that spinach goes down alarmingly when being cooked, so always buy at least twice as much as you imagine you will need.

8oz (225g) brown rice
2lb (900g) spinach, washed and roughly chopped
½ pint (300ml) vegetable stock
1 large onion, finely chopped

2–3 green peppers, seeded and sliced
1 clove garlic, crushed or finely chopped
2 teaspoons ground coriander
2 teaspoons ground cumin
¼ teaspoon cayenne pepper
sea salt
1 tablespoon tomato purée, or 2–3 fresh tomatoes,
skinned and chopped

PREPARATION TIME: 10–15 minutes
COOKING TIME: 25–30 minutes

Put the rice on to cook according to the instructions on
the packet. Add a little salt. When the rice has come to
the boil, start preparing the curry. First cook the spinach
by putting it in a saucepan without any extra water –
plenty will emerge as it cooks. Bring to the boil, cook for
about 10 minutes, then remove from the heat and drain
by pressing it hard to make it as dry as possible. Chop
very finely on a board. Heat vegetable stock in a
saucepan and add the onion, peppers, garlic, spices and
salt. Cook on a medium heat until the onion and peppers
are soft – about 10 minutes. Stir in the spinach and tomato purée or fresh chopped tomatoes, and continue to
cook for another 2 minutes. Serve at once with the rice.

Root Vegetable Curry

This is a very tasty and filling dish for winter, and will satisfy the hungriest eater.

8oz (225g) brown rice
1½ pints (990ml) vegetable stock
8oz (225g) turnips, peeled and cubed
8oz (225g) potatoes, peeled and cubed
8oz (225g) carrots, sliced
1 teaspoon ground turmeric
1 teaspoon ground cumin
1 teaspoon ground coriander
1 teaspoon garam masala
½ teaspoon cayenne pepper
2 bay leaves
2 cloves garlic, crushed or finely chopped
approx ½ teaspoon sea salt
2 tablespoons chopped coriander leaves (optional)

PREPARATION TIME 25–30 minutes
COOKING TIME: 40 minutes

Put the rice on to cook according to the instructions on the packet. When it is simmering, start the curry. Heat about ¼ pint (150ml) of the vegetable stock in a large saucepan and add the vegetables and spices. Stir over a medium heat for about 5 minutes, then bring to the boil. Add the rest of the stock, the bay leaves, garlic and salt. Lower the heat, cover and simmer for about 20 minutes or until the potatoes are done. Add the coriander, if using, then serve with the rice.

Cauliflower Curry

Cauliflowers lend themselves extremely well to curries and this one is colourful as well as tasty.

8oz (225g) brown rice
½ pint (300ml) vegetable stock
1 clove garlic, crushed
1 teaspoon ground cumin
1 teaspoon ground coriander
1 teaspoon grated fresh ginger root, or ¼ teaspoon powdered ginger
1 teaspoon ground turmeric
sea salt to taste
1 large onion, finely chopped
1 cauliflower, cut into small florets. Discard any tough-looking stalks
1 tablespoon tomato purée
4 large tomatoes, skinned and sliced

PREPARATION TIME: 10 minutes
COOKING TIME: about 30 minutes

Put the rice on to cook according to the instructions on the packet. When it has been simmering for 5 minutes, begin the curry. Heat half the vegetable stock in a large saucepan and add the garlic, spices, salt, onion and cauliflower. Stir over a medium heat for 5 minutes, then add the remaining stock and the tomato purée. Bring to the boil, then lower the heat, cover and simmer for 15 minutes. Just before serving, add the skinned and sliced tomatoes and serve at once with the rice.

CHINESE-STYLE DISHES

Chinese cookery lends itself very easily to the anti-cellulite regime, so long as you always stir-fry in stock rather than in any kind of oil. The secret of successful Chinese cookery is to chop up the vegetables very fine-ly and prepare the sauce beforehand, as this is a very quick method of cooking and you need to have all the ingredients to hand. Don't worry if you haven't got a wok; a large non-stick frying pan or saucepan will do. Although this method of cookery is very quick and easy, it does need constant attention.

Chinese-style anti-cellulite cookery has a sophisticat-ed taste and is more suitable for adults than children. I discovered it when I was trying to work out interesting dishes to keep me on my anti-cellulite diet, and found it a real taste sensation – so much cleaner and fresher-tasting than the kind of Chinese dishes, heavily reliant on oil and monosodium glutamate, that one finds in some Chinese restaurants.

Broccoli with Bamboo Shoots and Water Chestnuts

for the rice:
8oz (225g) brown rice
4 cups water (or twice as much as the rice)
1 teaspoon sea salt

for the sauce:
1 tablespoon vegetable stock
1 teaspoon cornflour
2 tablespoons dry sherry
1 tablespoon low-salt soy sauce

½ cup vegetable stock
8oz (225g) broccoli, finely chopped
2 tablespoons bean sprouts
1 clove garlic, crushed
1 teaspoon grated fresh ginger
1 small tin water chestnuts, finely sliced
1 small tin bamboo shoots

PREPARATION TIME: 10 minutes at most
COOKING TIME: 25–35 minutes, depending on rice

Put the rice and water in a saucepan, add salt and bring to the boil. Then cover and simmer (do not stir) for about 25 minutes Once the rice is simmering, make sure all the vegetables are ready, then make the sauce by mixing all the ingredients together in a bowl. Set aside.

Heat the stock in a large non-stick saucepan and stir-fry the broccoli, bean sprouts, garlic and ginger for 3 minutes. Lower the heat to medium and add the water chestnuts and bamboo shoots. Stir-fry for 2 minutes then add the sauce. Turn down the heat and simmer for 2 minutes. Serve immediately with the rice.

Braised Vegetables with Chinese Noodles

This is a highly sophisticated dish, suitable for dinner parties. It is especially suitable for anybody who is on a low-salt, low-fat or low-carbohydrate diet for any reason – good for slimmers and those who have to watch their food intake for health reasons.

for the sauce
2 tablespoons dry sherry
1 tablespoon soy sauce
1 tablespoon vegetable stock
1 teaspoon cornflour
8oz (225g) noodles – if using the Chinese noodles in compressed squares, allow 1 square per person

8 fl oz (250ml) vegetable stock
4oz (125g) mangetout peas, stems and strings
removed
8oz (225g) Chinese or white cabbage, shredded
8oz (225g) mushrooms, finely chopped
2 medium carrots, finely chopped
2 shallots or small onions, finely chopped
1 small green pepper, seeded and sliced
1 small red pepper, seeded and sliced
4oz (125g) beansprouts
1 tablespoon sesame seeds, roasted. (You can dry-
roast sesame seeds by stirring them for 1–2 minutes
in a pan on a high heat. Keep stirring, or they will
stick and burn.)

PREPARATION TIME: 15 minutes
COOKING TIME: 10 minutes

First, make the sauce by mixing together all the ingredients in a bowl. Set aside. Cook the noodles according
to the instructions on the packet. Heat the stock in a
large non-stick pan. When it is bubbling gently, add the
mangetout, cabbage, mushrooms, carrots, shallots and
peppers and stir-fry on a high heat for 3 minutes. Add the
beansprouts and stir-fry for 1 minute, then add the sauce,
lower the heat and simmer for 2 minutes. Add the roasted sesame seeds and serve immediately with the noodles.

Stir-Fried Rice and Vegetables

This Chinese dish will appeal to all tastes, including the faddy ones of many children. It has such a wonderful flavour that most people find they want to come back for more.

3 tablespoons vegetable stock
2 cloves garlic, crushed
1 tablespoon grated fresh ginger root, or ½ teaspoon powdered ginger
3 shallots or small onions, finely chopped
3 medium carrots, finely chopped
1 green pepper, seeded and sliced
1 red pepper, seeded and sliced
8oz (225g) broccoli, finely chopped
2oz (50g) bean sprouts
1 tablespoon soy sauce
2 tablespoons dry sherry
8oz (225g) cooked brown rice
freshly ground black pepper

PREPARATION TIME: 10 minutes
COOKING TIME: 10 minutes

Heat the stock in a large non-stick frying pan and stir-fry garlic, ginger and shallots for 2 minutes. Add the carrots, green and red peppers, broccoli and bean sprouts and stir-fry, lowering the heat slightly, for another 3 minutes. Add the soy sauce and dry sherry, stirring all the time, then add the cooked brown rice and continue to stir-fry until heated right through. Season with pepper and serve immediately.

Brown Rice and Carrots

I'm always falling back on this dish, which is easy and highly nutritious. It's also a good recipe if you have leftover cooked rice.

2–3 tablespoons vegetable stock
1 medium onion, finely chopped
8oz (225g) carrots, grated
2–3 courgettes, diced – or you could use 3-4 large
flat mushrooms
8oz (225g) brown rice, cooked
sea salt and freshly ground black pepper
2 tablespoons chopped fresh parsley
3 tablespoons sesame seeds

PREPARATION TIME: about 5 minutes
COOKING TIME: 10 minutes

Heat the vegetable stock in a large saucepan and stir-fry the onion and grated carrots for a few minutes until soft. Add the courgettes and continue cooking for a few more minutes, stirring all the time. Lower the heat, add the rice and stir in. Add the seasoning, parsley and sesame seeds. When all is heated through, serve with a mixed or green salad. Creamed spinach goes well with this dish, and adds welcome dark-green colour, especially if you use mushrooms.

COOKING WITH TOFU

A totally tasteless cheese-like white block in its natural state, tofu is a cellulite-shifter's delight. It is low in calories, dairy-free, highly nutritious, and blends in well with many kinds of food.

Tofu is easily available at every healthfood shop, it is cheap and versatile and can increasingly be found in supermarkets. It can be used in both savoury and sweet dishes instead of cheese and dairy products.

Tofu-Topped Vegetables

This dish, which is quick and easy to prepare, is popular at dinner parties. I cook it often, and it has been pronounced delicious by people who have never heard of tofu and who would probably turn their noses up at it if you told them what it was. (I'm thinking of the typical meat-and-two-veg unreconstructed male, who affects to despise 'healthy' food.)

1lb (450g) fresh spinach, or use frozen leaf spinach
½ cup vegetable stock
12oz (350g) white cabbage, shredded
2 leeks, cleaned and chopped
3–4 courgettes, diced
3–4 carrots, diced
2 cloves garlic, crushed
1 teaspoon sea salt
freshly ground black pepper
2 packs tofu – firm, if possible, not silken
3 tablespoons tahini
juice 1 lemon
1 teaspoon soy sauce
4 tablespoons natural low-fat yoghurt, or use
natural soya yoghurt
¼ teaspoon cayenne pepper
2oz (50g) wholemeal breadcrumbs (optional)

PREPARATION TIME: 15 minutes
COOKING TIME: 45–50 minutes

Preheat the oven to 350ºF, 180ºC, gas mark 4.

Cook the spinach until tender. It's easy to cook spinach – the real problem is getting it free from grit, which is why lazy cooks (like me) tend to use the frozen variety. Fresh, just-washed spinach does not need water adding; just put it all in a pan, bring to the boil and cook over a medium heat for about 5 minutes. You'll be amazed at how quickly fresh spinach reduces.

Heat the stock in a large non-stick pan and stir-fry the cabbage and leeks for 1–2 minutes. Cover, lower the heat and simmer for 4–5 minutes more. Add the courgettes and carrots and stir-fry for 4–5 minutes over a medium heat, then add the garlic and cook for 4 more minutes. Add the cooked spinach to the pan with the sea salt and pepper. Remove from the heat and transfer the contents to a large casserole dish.

In a liquidizer, combine the tofu, tahini, lemon juice, soy sauce, yoghurt and cayenne pepper and liquidize until smooth. Pour over the vegetables and top with the breadcrumbs, if using. Bake for about 35 minutes or until it is slightly browned and bubbling gently.

Serve with salad. Jacket potatoes (see page 261) go well with this dish.

Tofu Shepherd's Pie

This is such an improvement on the traditional version, and it is popular with all age groups and even fussy eaters.

½ cup vegetable stock
1 onion, finely chopped
8oz (225g) mushrooms, chopped
1 green pepper, seeded and sliced
2 large carrots, finely chopped

6 tomatoes, skinned, or 14oz (400g) tin tomatoes, chopped
1 bay leaf
2 heaped teaspoons fresh chopped basil, or
½ teaspoon dried
1 pack Morinaga or Tofeata tofu
sea salt and freshly ground black pepper to taste
1lb (450g) mashed potatoes (do not mash them with butter, cream or milk)

PREPARATION TIME: about 15 minutes
COOKING TIME: 45 minutes

Preheat the oven to 375°F, 190°C, gas mark 5.

Heat the stock in a non-stick pan, add the onion and stir-fry for 2 minutes. Add the mushrooms, green pepper and carrots and continue to stir-fry over a medium heat for about 3 minutes, then add the tomatoes, bay leaf and basil. Cover and simmer for about 15 minutes.

Chop or break up the tofu and add to the vegetable mixture, stirring all the time. Add the sea salt and black pepper, then turn the mixture into a large casserole and top with the mashed potatoes. Bake in the oven for 20 minutes or until the potatoes are lightly browned.

Serve with a green salad; it doesn't need anything else.

PULSES

Pulses – lentils, black-eyed beans, haricot beans, kidney beans, even baked beans if they are sugar-free – are marvellous foods for those wishing to be rid of cellulite. They provide complex carbohydrates and are nutritionally satisfying, tasty and versatile. I used to soak pulses overnight, but now I've become rather lazy and tend to use those pulses that can be cooked from start to finish in about half an hour, or I use tins. Chick peas and kidney beans tin well, and in recipes it is impossible to tell the difference. Always rinse tinned pulses in filtered water before using, as they tend to be preserved in brine.

However, as it is always useful – and cheaper – to have stocks of dried pulses, this is how to cook them by the quick-soak method rather than soaking overnight. Allow 8oz (225g) pulses for four people. They will swell up to twice their size when cooked.

Haricot beans Put 8oz (225g) beans in a saucepan with 1½ pints (900ml) water, cover and bring to the boil. Simmer for 2 minutes, then turn off the heat. Leave to soak for 2–3 hours, then bring to the boil again, reduce heat and simmer for 2 hours until tender.

Butter beans Soak 8oz (225g) beans overnight in plenty of cold water. The next day, drain, rinse, then put in a pan with 2 pints (1.2l) fresh water. Bring to the boil, reduce heat, and simmer for 3 hours or until tender.

Chick peas Put 8oz (225g) chick peas in a saucepan with 2 pints (1.2l) water, cover and bring to the boil. Simmer for 2 minutes, then turn off the heat and leave to soak for 3 hours. Bring to the boil again and simmer for another 3 hours or until they are very tender.

Black-eyed beans These have the advantage of cooking very quickly without pre-soaking. Bring 8oz (225g) blackeyed beans to the boil in 1 pint (600ml) water, then reduce heat, cover and simmer for 30 minutes or until tender.

Kidney beans These are difficult to cook properly, which is why I always buy tins and drain off the fluid. But for 8oz (225g) beans you need 1 pint (600ml) water. Put the beans in a saucepan with the water and bring to the boil. Cover and simmer for 2 minutes. Let stand for about 3 hours, then bring to the boil again and boil hard for 10 minutes. Reduce the heat and simmer for 1 hour, or until extremely tender.

Aduki beans Put 8oz (225g) aduki beans into a saucepan with 1 pint (600ml) water and bring to the boil. Simmer for 2 minutes, turn off the heat and leave to stand for 1 hour. Bring to the boil again and simmer for 1 hour or until tender.

Red and brown lentils These cook quickly and do not need pre-soaking. Using twice as much water as lentils, bring to the boil and simmer, covered, until cooked and mushy. Red lentils take 30 minutes at most, and brown ones about 45 minutes. Check every now and again that the water has not evaporated, as burned lentils are horrible. While cooking, they can be flavoured with a bay leaf.

Note: if you have a pressure cooker, you can cut down the cooking time considerably. Cook according to the instructions for your model.

For all beans, sea salt can be added towards the end of the cooking time. This takes out some of the 'windiness' associated with beans.

Lentil Shepherd's Pie

¾ pint (450ml) vegetable stock
1 large onion, finely chopped
1 stick celery, chopped
6oz (175g) red lentils
½ teaspoon yeast extract
¼ teaspoon fresh thyme or pinch dried
¼ teaspoon fresh sage or pinch dried
6oz (175g) carrots, grated
1lb (450g) potatoes
1 bay leaf
sea salt and freshly ground black pepper
a little low-fat yoghurt or fromage frais

PREPARATION TIME: about 20 minutes
COOKING TIME: about 45 minutes

Heat about 2 tablespoons of the stock in a large non-stick frying pan and stir-fry the onion and celery for about 2 minutes. Add the lentils, remaining stock, yeast extract, thyme, sage and grated carrots and bring to the boil. Simmer for 30 minutes. Meanwhile, scrub potatoes, cut into 2 inch (5cm) pieces, place in a pan with the bay leaf and cover with water. Add 1 teaspoon sea salt and bring to the boil, then simmer for 25 minutes or until tender. Drain, and mash with freshly ground black pepper and a little low-fat yoghurt or fromage frais. Place the lentil mixture in a pie dish and top with the potato. Heat under the grill for about 5 minutes.

Serve with steamed spinach, broccoli or cabbage, or a green salad.

Brown Lentils and Buckwheat Spaghetti

This is an all-time favourite with my family. Most children love it, and don't even realize that there is no meat in it. The only drawback is that it takes rather a long time to cook.

8oz (225g) brown lentils
1 pint (600ml) water
2 bay leaves
sea salt and freshly ground black pepper
1½ pints (900ml) vegetable stock
1 onion, chopped

1 clove garlic, crushed
4 large carrots, chopped
2 sticks celery, chopped
1 dessertspoon tomato purée
4oz (125g) mushrooms, chopped
2–3 tablespoons chopped fresh parsley

PREPARATION TIME: 20 minutes
COOKING TIME: about 1½ hours

Preheat the oven to 400ºF, 200ºC, gas mark 6.

Put the lentils into a pan with the water, and bay leaves and seasoning. Bring to the boil, cover, then lower the heat and simmer for about 45 minutes, making sure it does not boil dry. You may need to taste from time to time to see if the lentils are cooked – if there is a trace of hardness they need longer.

Meanwhile heat about ¼ pint (150ml) of the stock in a large, non-stick frying pan and stir in the onion and garlic. Stir-fry for about 5 minutes over a medium heat. Stir in the carrots and celery and cook for a few minutes more, then add the tomato purée and the rest of the stock. Bring to the boil, then add the mushrooms, cooked lentils and parsley. Season, then lower the heat and simmer for about 45 minutes. About 10 minutes before the sauce is ready, cook the buckwheat spaghetti according to instructions. Serve topped with the lentil sauce.

Vegetable Casserole

This is a really simple casserole which makes a good
weekday supper dish.

  8oz (275g) brown lentils
  3–4 medium carrots, chopped
  2 sticks celery, chopped
  2 onions, finely chopped
  1 heaped teaspoon each chopped fresh sage and
  thyme, or ½ teaspoon each dried
  1 large cooking apple, cored and chopped
  sea salt and freshly ground black pepper
  ¾ pint (450ml) vegetable stock
  1 tablespoon oatflakes

  PREPARATION TIME: 10 minutes
  COOKING TIME: about 45 minutes

Preheat the oven to 350°F, 180°C, gas mark 4.

Put all the ingredients except the oatflakes into a
casserole and cover completely with vegetable stock.
Sprinkle over the oatflakes, cover with a tight-fitting
lid and bake in the oven for about 45 minutes or until
completely cooked.

Lentil and Swede Bake

Many people turn up their noses at swedes, but cooked this way they are delicious and tasty, and quite unlike the mashed tasteless swedes we remember from school dinners.

8oz (225g) red lentils
1 pint (600ml) water
2 bay leaves
sea salt and freshly ground black pepper
8oz (225g) swede, grated
¼ pint (150ml) vegetable stock
1 medium onion, chopped
2 sticks celery, chopped
about ⅛ nutmeg, grated
2 tablespoons chopped fresh parsley
a little olive oil
4 tablespoons wholemeal breadcrumbs

PREPARATION TIME: about 20 minutes
COOKING TIME: 1 hour 20 minutes

Preheat the oven to 400°F, 200°C, gas mark 6.

Put the lentils into a saucepan with the water, bay leaves and seasoning. Bring to the boil, cover and simmer gently for about 40 minutes. Mix in the grated swede and cook for another 10 minutes, by which time all the water should be absorbed. Remove from the heat.

While the lentils are cooking, heat the vegetable stock in a separate pan and cook the onion and celery over a gentle heat until tender – about 15 minutes. Mix into the lentil and swede purée, adding the nutmeg and parsley. Season again to taste, then transfer to an oiled casserole dish – just smear a little olive oil over the surface with a paper towel – and sprinkle over the wholemeal breadcrumbs. Bake in the oven for 30 minutes.

Kidney Bean Casserole

This is a very warming and filling winter dish. As it contains chillies, it is also quite hot. If you are cooking this dish for children or people who don't like very spicy food, omit the chillies and instead use 1 dessert-spoon paprika.

8oz (225g) red kidney beans, or 14oz (400g) tin
1 pint (600ml) water, if using dried beans
1lb (450g) tomatoes, skinned and sliced
sea salt and freshly ground black pepper
2 large red peppers, seeded and sliced
2 medium onions, sliced
1 clove garlic, crushed
2 fresh red chillies, seeded and finely chopped, or
2 dried red chillies
2 teaspoons paprika

PREPARATION TIME: about 15 minutes
COOKING TIME: if using tinned beans, 1½ hours;
otherwise, about 2½ hours.

If using dried kidney beans, cook them according to
the instructions on page 280. Preheat the oven to 325°F,
160°C, gas mark 3.

Layer half the tomatoes in a large casserole, season
well, then add a layer of peppers, onions and garlic,
chillies and paprika. Put in all the beans, followed by a
second layer of peppers, onions and garlic, with the
remaining tomatoes on top. Season again. Cover the
casserole and bake in the oven for about 1½ hours.
Serve with brown rice and a green salad.

Black-eyed Beans with Mixed Vegetables

A very filling and tasty dish. Black-eyed beans cook
very quickly and have a creamy taste.

8oz (225g) black-eyed beans
1 pint (600ml) water
about ½ pint (300ml) vegetable stock
1 large onion, sliced
1 clove garlic, crushed
12oz (350g) courgettes, sliced
12oz (350g) tomatoes, skinned and sliced
12oz (350g) flat mushrooms, chopped

1 green pepper, seeded and sliced
sea salt and freshly ground black pepper
1 tablespoon mixed fresh herbs, or 1 teaspoon dried

PREPARATION TIME: around 15 minutes
COOKING TIME: 35–40 minutes

Put the black-eyed beans into a saucepan with the water and bring to the boil. Reduce heat and simmer until tender (about 30 minutes). Meanwhile, heat 2–3 tablespoons of the vegetable stock in a large saucepan and sweat the onions, garlic and courgettes over a medium heat for 5 minutes. Add the remaining vegetables and stock and bring to the boil. Season, add the herbs, then lower the heat and simmer until the vegetables are cooked – about 15 minutes. When the black-eyed beans are ready, stir into the vegetable mixture and check the seasoning. Serve with a green salad and, if liked, jacket potatoes. Brown rice could also accompany this dish.

Vegetable Bake

3 medium onions, chopped
3–4 carrots, diced
2 large old potatoes, peeled and sliced
½ pint (300ml) vegetable stock
2 tablespoons chopped fresh mint, or 2 teaspoons dried

sea salt and freshly ground black pepper
1 tablespoon cold-pressed oil
2 cloves garlic, crushed
2 tablespoons sesame seeds

PREPARATION TIME: about 10 minutes
COOKING TIME: about 45 minutes

Preheat the oven to 400ºF, 200ºC, gas mark 6.

Put the onions, carrots, potatoes and vegetable stock into a saucepan. Bring to the boil, then lower the heat and simmer for about 15 minutes or until the vegetables are cooked.

Transfer the onions, carrots and any remaining stock to a lightly oiled casserole dish, mixing in the mint and seasoning well. Then arrange the potatoes on top. Brush the oil over the potatoes and sprinkle with the garlic and sesame seeds. Bake in the oven for about 30 minutes or until the potatoes turn golden-brown.

Vegetable Risotto

A colourful and easy dish, complete in itself, which will be popular with all the family.

8oz (225g) brown rice
1 large onion, finely chopped
1 clove garlic, crushed

3 tablespoons vegetable stock
1lb (450g) spinach, washed and chopped
8oz (225g) broccoli, chopped
corn from 1 corn on the cob, or use tinned corn
4oz (125g) cashews (*not* salted or roasted ones)
1 teaspoon fresh or ½ teaspoon dried rosemary
1 teaspoon fresh or ½ teaspoon dried tarragon
about ⅙ nutmeg, grated
pinch powdered cloves
1 tablespoon chopped fresh parsley
sea salt and freshly ground black pepper

PREPARATION TIME: 10 minutes
COOKING TIME: about 40 minutes

Cook the brown rice in lightly salted water. While the rice is simmering, sweat the onion and garlic for about 5 minutes in the vegetable stock over a medium heat. Add the spinach, broccoli, and corn, and stir-fry until the vegetables are tender. Do not allow to burn and stick to the pan. Dry-roast the cashews for a few minutes in a heavy pan over medium heat, stirring all the time.

When the rice is cooked, stir in the vegetables, cashews, herbs, cloves and parsley. Season to taste and heat through very gently. Serve immediately.

Spinach and Noodles

This is extremely quick and easy, provides a fully balanced meal and is enormously popular, in my experience.

8oz (225g) wholemeal noodles or wholemeal macaroni
2lb (900g) spinach, washed and chopped
4oz (125g) cashew nuts
1 sprig rosemary, finely chopped, or ½ teaspoon dried rosemary
about ⅛ nutmeg, grated
sea salt and freshly ground black pepper
4 tablespoons natural low-fat yoghurt, or plain soya yoghurt
4 tomatoes, skinned and sliced

PREPARATION TIME: about 10 minutes
COOKING TIME: 15 minutes

Cook the noodles or macaroni according to the instructions on the packet. At the same time, cook the spinach for about 10 minutes in only the water that is left after washing. Dry-roast the cashews over a medium heat, stirring until they start to turn brown, then remove at once. Remove the spinach from the saucepan, drain and chop finely. Transfer back to the saucepan, and add the rosemary, nutmeg, salt and pepper. Stir over a low heat for 2 minutes, making sure it does not burn, then add the yoghurt and stir thoroughly until completely heated through. By this time the noodles should be ready. Drain and transfer to a heated serving dish and pile the spinach mixture on top. Arrange the tomatoes over the spinach and serve at once.

Carrot Purée

This is an easy and tasty way of cooking big, old carrots. Serve with jacket potatoes, brown rice or as an accompanying vegetable to a bake or casserole.

¼ pint (150ml) water
4 large carrots, sliced
1½oz (40g) oatbran or finely milled oats
2 fl oz (50ml) skimmed milk or soya milk
sea salt and freshly ground black pepper to taste
½ teaspoon ground cinnamon
about ⅛ nutmeg, grated
2 tablespoons chopped mixed nuts – brazils, cashews, hazels

PREPARATION TIME: 6–7 minutes
COOKING TIME: 40 minutes

Preheat the oven to 375ºF, 190ºC, gas mark 5.

Bring the water to the boil, add the carrots and cook quickly until tender – about 10 minutes. Transfer the carrots plus their cooking water to a liquidizer and blend until smooth with all the remaining ingredients except the nuts. Check the seasoning, then transfer to an ovenproof dish, scatter the chopped mixed nuts on top and bake in the oven for 30 minutes.

Special Burgers

Even vegetable burgers can be cooked without using oil or fat. These burgers have a taste all of their own and are delicious and filling. Children love them as much as adults do, and they have the added advantage that they are not soaked in fat, like ordinary burgers. They are also extremely easy to make.

8oz (225g) red lentils
1 bay leaf
sea salt and freshly ground black pepper
4oz (125g) mixed nuts (not peanuts), ground
2oz (50g) sunflower seeds, ground
1 medium onion or 2 shallots, chopped and sweated
    until soft in a little vegetable stock. Or you could
    use finely chopped celery instead
1 tablespoon oatmeal
1 dessertspoon chopped fresh sage or 1 teaspoon
    dried

few celery seeds (optional)
a little oil for brushing burgers

PREPARATION TIME: 10 minutes
COOKING TIME: 1 hour 10 minutes

Preheat the oven to 400°F, 200°C, gas mark 6.

Put the lentils in a saucepan with the bay leaf, a little salt and pepper and twice as much water as lentils. Bring to the boil, then reduce heat, cover and simmer until a purée is formed – about 30 minutes. The purée should be fairly mushy as the burgers will dry out when they are cooked. Check once or twice during cooking that the mixture has not started to stick to the bottom of the pan. When the lentils are cooked, remove the bay leaf.

Mix all the ingredients (except the oil) with the lentil purée in a large mixing bowl and form into burgers. This mixture will make 4–6, depending on size. Lightly oil a baking tray and brush each burger with a little olive or cold-pressed vegetable oil, if you like. This is not essential, but stops the tops from becoming too 'biscuity'. Bake in the oven for 40 minutes, or until slightly browned. Serve with quark or low-fat yoghurt (other members of the family can have sour cream, if they like, or tomato ketchup) and a large salad.

NUT LOAVES

Nut loaves are the vegetarian equivalent of roasts. They are quite time-consuming to prepare and cook, but good for special occasions. All nut loaves can be made in advance and then frozen until needed.

Nut savouries can be made with a huge variety of different nuts, but whatever quantity of nuts you use, you should have an equal amount of cooked brown rice, potatoes or breadcrumbs to act as 'backing'. Otherwise the nuts are too dry and indigestible. You also need flavouring – onions, garlic, shallots, mushrooms, courgettes – and some liquid so that it all coalesces together before you bake. Most nut loaves and savouries take about 40 minutes to bake in a moderate oven. Don't overbake, otherwise they will be dry and biscuity.

Simple Brazil Nut Roast

This is one of the easiest to make. As with all nut loaves, it is very filling. You can use other nuts, such as hazels or cashews, in this basic recipe.

1 large onion, finely chopped
4oz (125g) carrots, grated
about 3 tablespoons vegetable stock
4oz (125g) brazil nuts, finely milled

4oz (125g) wholemeal breadcrumbs
1 teaspoon chopped fresh sage or rosemary or
¼ teaspoon dried
sea salt and freshly ground black pepper
3 level tablespoons soya flour
1 tablespoon sesame seeds

PREPARATION TIME: 15 minutes
COOKING TIME: about 45 minutes

Preheat the oven to 350°F, 180°C, gas mark 4.

Sweat the onion and carrots over a medium heat in 2–3 tablespoons vegetable stock for 5 minutes. Add the nuts, breadcrumbs, herbs, seasonings and flour. If the mixture is too dry, add a little more vegetable stock. It should be sticky but not runny. Press into a 1lb (450g) loaf tin and sprinkle with the sesame seeds. Bake in the oven for 30–40 minutes. Serve with salad.

Hazelnut and Tomato Bake

This is a variation on the nut loaf and has been a favourite in my family for many years. It is particularly popular with teenagers.

2–3 tablespoons vegetable stock
1 medium onion, finely chopped
1 clove garlic, crushed

1lb (450g) tomatoes, skinned and chopped
½ tablespoon tomato purée
6oz (175g) hazelnuts, ground
8oz (225g) mashed potato
1 tablespoon chopped fresh parsley
1 teaspoon fresh or ¼ teaspoon dried basil
a little olive oil for greasing dish
grated rind ¼ lemon
sea salt and freshly ground black pepper

PREPARATION TIME: 10 minutes
COOKING TIME: 40-55 minutes

Preheat the oven to 350°F, 180°C, gas mark 4.

Heat the stock in a large saucepan and cook the onion and garlic for about 5 minutes until softened. Add the tomatoes and boil until reduced in quantity and completely mushy – about 5–10 minutes. Add the tomato purée, remove from the heat and stir in all the remaining ingredients except the olive oil, mixing well. Grease an ovenproof dish with a little olive oil, press in the mixture and bake in the oven for 30–40 minutes. Serve with plain yoghurt and a green salad. This dish is very filling, and a little goes a long way.

Chapter 20

Fish and Meat Main Courses

This section has been contributed by aromatherapist Frances Clifford, who helped me to get rid of my cellulite.

Meat and fish, says Frances, have very little place in any successful cellulite-shedding regime. The reason is that both these foods clog up the system and putrefy quickly once in the bowel. Also, they do not combine successfully with carbohydrates in the digestive system. Therefore they should be eaten only infrequently – once a week for chicken or other meat, say Sunday lunch, and twice a week for fish. Do not eat animal protein more often than this while you are trying to lose cellulite. Some people do feel better if they eat fish and meat once in a while to gain their full vitamin and amino-acid complement. (Most vegetarians seem to make up the lack without any trouble at all, and few vegetarians are ever found to be grossly deficient in their diet. In fact, it is more likely to be the meat eaters who are deficient.)

When buying meat, make sure it is locally reared, fresh and unprocessed. Do not buy meats that have been extensively processed, smoked, or contain preservatives or additives. Avoid tinned meats, ready-prepared meat meals, bought meat sauces and such dubious delights as hamburgers, fried chicken, doner kebabs and sausages.

Buy meat from a small, independent butcher or from an organization such as the Real Meat Company. Their address is East Hill Farm, Heytesbury, near Warminster, Wilts, BA12 oHR. At the point of sale, meat should be displayed in such a way that air can circulate. The fat should be of a white or creamy colour, with a matt finish. You may find that additive-free, organically produced meat is a paler colour than you have been used to, but that is an indication that no dyes have been added. All meat you buy should smell fresh.

Fish should also be bought as close to its source as possible. Fresh fish is bright-eyed, bright-skinned and not slimy-looking or strange-smelling. Wet-fish counters have now appeared in many supermarkets and these have a quick turnover. Alternatively, find an independent fishmonger where you can check that the fish is freshly caught.

When cooking meat or fish the anti-cellulite way, do not fry or barbecue as very hot cooking oil releases free radicals. It is better to 'dry-roast' meat – that is, put it in a covered pot or casserole with seasonings, and cook on a very low heat (275°F, 140°C, gas mark 1) for several hours. If you have a crockpot, you will find this invaluable, but whatever you do, never fry the meat in oil first.

Small pieces of meat can be grilled under a low to medium heat. The use of aromatic herbs and spices improves the smell of cooking meat and also stimulates the flow of vital digestive juices.

Remember that human beings are not really designed to eat meat, as our colons are too long. A heavy meat diet causes constant putrefaction in the colon and a steady process of autointoxication which eventually adds to the cellulite load. You may also experience feelings of lethargy, bloating and heaviness after eating too much meat or fish – hence the time-honoured nap after Sunday lunch. Frances recommends that if you ever feel heavy after eating meat you should go completely vegetarian for a while.

For those who feel they need some meat or fish in their diet (or who are reluctant to give it up completely) Frances recommends a ninety per cent vegetarian, ten per cent meat or fish diet. This is completely adequate – nobody needs more animal protein than this. Relegate meat and fish to bit-part players instead of assigning them the leading role in your cookery.

Frances attributes her own abundant good health to a diet that contains very few animal products of any kind.

These are Frances's favourite anti-cellulite fish and meat recipes – the ones she recommends to her patients who wish to be rid of their cellulite deposits.

Lemon-baked Plaice

1–2 fillets plaice per person
grated rind ½ lemon and 2 teaspoons lemon juice
per fillet
sea salt and freshly ground black pepper
2 dessertspoons mixed fresh herbs – thyme,
marjoram, parsley, oregano, for example – or
¼ teaspoon mixed dried herbs per fillet
lemon wedges and parsley sprigs to garnish

PREPARATION TIME: 10 minutes
COOKING TIME: 40–50 minutes

Preheat the oven to 325ºF, 170ºC, gas mark 3.

Season each fillet with lemon rind, salt and pepper.
Roll each one up and secure with a cocktail stick or
skewer. Pack the prepared fillets into a casserole, sprinkle over the mixed herbs, cover with the remaining
lemon juice and rind, and cover with a lid.

Cook for about 40–50 minutes, or until the plaice is
completely white and flakes easily. When ready, lift out
with a fish slice onto a warmed serving dish. Garnish
with the lemon wedges and parsley. Serve with a
mixed green salad, steamed mangetout and new baby
carrots or baby corn.

Note: This recipe can be adapted to any kind of flat fish.

Dinner Party Salmon

1 bay leaf per steak
1 salmon steak per person. Buy wild salmon if
possible
about ½ teaspoon extra-virgin olive oil per steak
sea salt and freshly ground black pepper
juice ½ lemon or 1 teaspoon dry martini per steak
1 dessertspoon chopped chives or parsley per
salmon steak

PREPARATION TIME: 10 minutes
COOKING TIME: about 20 minutes

Lightly oil a large grill pan with olive oil. Arrange the
bay leaves in the pan and place 1 salmon steak on each.
Brush the steaks with the olive oil and season with salt
and pepper. Cook gently under the grill – the flame
should not be turned up high and the steaks must not
be allowed to char – to allow natural oils to be released
and also so that the bay leaf aroma penetrates each
steak.

After about 20 minutes, or when the fish is flaky,
pour over the lemon juice or dry martini and replace for
a maximum of 1 minute under the grill. Put the steaks
on a hot serving plate with the cooking juices, and garnish with chopped chives or parsley. Serve with tossed
green salad and mixed steamed vegetables.

This dish can be kept warm in the oven for 30 minutes, on a very low heat, if kept well covered. This gives time for a starter.

Note: this recipe can be used for any fish steaks.

Aromatic Pot-Roast Chicken

Organically reared, free-range chicken smells quite delicious when cooking and produces relatively few juices compared to mass-produced birds that have been plumped up with water and preservatives.

1 organically reared chicken, corn-fed if possible
2–4 garlic cloves, peeled and halved
2 lemon halves, or 1 onion, peeled, with up to 10 cloves pressed into it
extra-virgin olive oil
sea salt and freshly ground black pepper
1 teaspoon dried or 1 dessertspoon fresh tarragon or rosemary
lemon wedges, fresh herbs, raw onion rings to garnish

PREPARATION TIME: 15–20 minutes
COOKING TIME: 1½–1¾ hours

Preheat the oven to 400°F, 200°C, gas mark 6.

Prepare the chicken by rinsing in cold water inside and out, then dry with a piece of kitchen towel roll.

Discard the giblets. Using a sharp pointed knife, make 4–8 deep slits in the fleshiest part of the chicken – thigh or breast – and push the garlic halves well down into these.

Put the lemon halves or the onion inside the chicken. Smear the upper part of the chicken with olive oil and put into a casserole. Season with salt and pepper and tarragon or rosemary. Cover with a lid and cook for 30–45 minutes, then reduce the heat to 300°F, 150°C, gas mark 2 and cook for 1 further hour. Test by sticking a knife in the thigh. If the juices run clear, the chicken is cooked.

To serve, place the chicken on a preheated dish. Remove the lemon or onion and pour the cooking juices over and around the bird. Garnish with lemon wedges and fresh tarragon or a few raw onion rings and sprigs of rosemary.

Serve with steamed carrots and broccoli, and a green salad.

Chicken cooked in this way is also very good cold.

Chicken Roll

This is very similar to the previous recipe and uses the same ingredients. Ask your butcher to bone the chicken for you.

Prepare on a chopping board a mixture of chopped or crushed garlic cloves, grated lemon rind and green herbs, such as parsley or thyme. Spread the chicken out with the inside facing up, and scatter this mixture all over. Season with sea salt and freshly ground black pepper.

Roll the chicken up carefully and use skewers to keep it in a roll shape. Pot roast as before but increase slow cooking time by 30 minutes, as there are no bones to conduct the heat.

This dish is also very good cold.

Lamb

This is the only other 'everyday' meat that Frances recommends to her patients and even this should be eaten very seldom (about once or twice a month maximum) as it is high in fat and can be indigestible if you are trying to refine your diet. English lamb in season – Easter and early summer – is best because it has been subjected to less handling than imported lamb.

Lamb should be cooked using the 'pot roast' method as with chicken, and can be flavoured with lemon or rosemary. Garlic can be inserted into the meat if desired, and the joint can be seasoned with sea salt and freshly ground pepper.

Game Birds

Game eaten in season is very good and makes a welcome change from other forms of flesh protein. Always try to ensure that the game is wild and has been shot on the wing. Wild birds are lean and should be cooked slowly to preserve moisture. Duck, guinea fowl, pheasant and quail are all good and may be grilled or spit-roasted. Brush first with a very small amount of olive oil.

Pigeon are best braised on a bed of mixed vegetables, such as leeks and carrots, with a little red wine. Juniper berries are the best seasoning for game birds. Consult standard cookery books for game bird ideas, but always use the pot roast method of cooking. Never fry or barbecue.

Chapter 21

Puddings

Many people imagine that anyone who is serious about shifting cellulite will have to forego puddings for ever. However, this is not quite true. Although double cream and huge slices of Black Forest gâteau are out – except for the very occasional indulgence – there are ways in which you can end a meal with something satisfyingly sweet. For many of us, life would be bleak indeed without any puddings.

Here are some desserts that will cheer you up and satisfy the longing for something sweet at the end of a meal, without encouraging the dread cellulite to return.

Apricot and Tofu Dessert

Yes, our old friend tofu comes to the rescue here. When testing the recipes for this book I asked two people who happened to be in the house at the time – my cleaning lady and a decorator – to try this dish.

Although initially suspicious they both, to their surprise, found that they enjoyed eating it, even though it contained unfamiliar ingredients. You can serve this dessert with confidence at a dinner party.

Although this dish is simple and quick to prepare, it has to be thought about several hours in advance if you are using dried apricots.

4–6oz (125–175g) dried Hunza apricots, soaked overnight and drained, or use the same quantity fresh apricots
1 pack tofu
juice ½ lemon
4 tablespoons raw sugar or organic honey
2 tablespoons low-fat natural yoghurt or plain soya yoghurt
3–4 tablespoons flaked almonds

PREPARATION TIME: 5 minutes
COOKING TIME: nil

Combine all the ingredients except the almonds in a liquidizer. Blend until smooth, then spoon into 4 glass dishes. Top with the almonds and chill.

Strawberries with Tofu

1lb (450g) strawberries (or you could use
raspberries)
1 pack tofu
¼ teaspoon natural vanilla essence
juice 1 lemon
4–5 tablespoons raw sugar or honey

PREPARATION TIME: 5 minutes
COOKING TIME: nil

Put most of the strawberries or raspberries in a liquidizer and blend with all the other ingredients until
smooth. Spoon into individual glass dishes and decorate with the remaining fruit. Chill before serving.

Tofu Cheesecake

Yes, you can have cheesecake – so long as you make it
like this. As it takes a long time to chill, it is best to make
it in the morning, or even the night before you need it.

¼ cup rolled oats
½oz (15g) desiccated coconut
½oz (15g) butter
1 pack tofu

2 tablespoons low-fat natural yoghurt
2 tablespoons raw sugar or organic honey
juice and rind ½ orange
½ teaspoon natural vanilla essence
2 teaspoons tahini
pinch sea salt
2–3 tablespoons organic honey
4 tablespoons water
½ teaspoon powdered agar-agar (vegetarian gelling agent, available from healthfood shops)
4oz (125g) fresh or frozen raspberries

PREPARATION TIME: 15 minutes
COOKING TIME: about 40 minutes

Preheat the oven to 350°F, 180°C, gas mark 4.

Mix the oats and coconut together in a bowl. Spread the butter over the bottom of an 8 inch (20cm) flan tin, then sprinkle the oat and coconut mixture over this. Press down and set aside. In a liquidizer, combine the tofu, yoghurt, sugar or honey, orange juice and rind, vanilla essence, tahini and salt. When thoroughly blended, pour into the flan case. In a small pan melt the honey in the water over a medium heat and stir in the agar-agar. Bring to the boil and simmer for about 1 minute. Remove from the heat, stir in the raspberries, and pour over the tofu mixture in the flan case. Bake in the oven for 35 minutes. Leave to cool, then chill for several hours before serving.

Fruit Purée with Muesli Topping

This can be served with nut cream or low-fat yoghurt. Use the tiny Hunza dried apricots. They look unappetizing when dried but are far tastier than the bright-orange, sulphured variety.

4oz (125g) dried Hunza apricots, soaked overnight
4oz (125g) sunflower seeds, ground
1 banana
1 apple
juice ½ lemon
¼ teaspoon organic honey

for the topping
4oz (125g) muesli base
2oz (50g) raisins
2oz (50g) flaked almonds
2oz (50g) sunflower seeds
2oz (50g) desiccated coconut (Or you could use Sunwheel 45 per cent fruit and nut de luxe muesli instead.)

PREPARATION TIME: 10 minutes
COOKING TIME: 5 minutes

Blend together in a liquidizer the apricots, sunflower seeds, banana, apple, lemon juice and honey, adding a little water if the mixture seems too stiff.

Toast the ingredients for the muesli topping under the grill until slightly browned. This will make it crunchy. Spread the topping over the purée and serve.

Baked Apples

This good old British standby makes a wonderful dessert for cellulite watchers.

1 large cooking apple per person, cored

to fill each apple:
½ tablespoon ground or finely chopped brazil nuts
1 tablespoon sultanas or currants
½ teaspoon ground cinnamon
½ teaspoon ground coriander

PREPARATION TIME: 5 minutes
COOKING TIME: 35 minutes

Preheat the oven to 350°F, 180°C, gas mark 4.

To prevent the apples exploding, cut a ring in the peel round the middle before baking. Stuff with the remaining ingredients then bake in the oven for 35 minutes. Serve with nut cream (see page 316), low-fat yoghurt or soya yoghurt.

Peaches with Sesame Seeds

This makes a change from the usual peaches and cream.
Use fresh peaches in season rather than tinned ones.

    5oz (150g) sesame seeds
    6oz (175g) raisins
    1 teaspoon ground cinnamon
    4 peaches
    1 dessertspoon dry sherry

PREPARATION TIME: 10 minutes
COOKING TIME: 25 minutes

Preheat the oven to 375°F, 190°C, gas mark 5.

Mix together the sesame seeds, raisins and cinnamon. Cut the peaches in half, remove the stones, and fill the holes with the sesame seed mixture. Place in an earthenware ovenproof dish, pour over the sherry and bake for 25 minutes, then serve.

Yoghurt Fool

This can be made with almost any kind of fruit, although soft fruits make the nicest yoghurt fools. You need never buy flavoured or sugared yoghurts again. Always buy the plain, low-fat variety and add your own flavourings.

2 punnets strawberries, raspberries, blackcurrants
or redcurrants
2 cartons low-fat yoghurt or plain soya yoghurt
teaspoon honey, or to taste
teaspoon natural vanilla essence
chopped nuts to serve (optional)

PREPARATION TIME: 5 minutes
COOKING TIME: nil

Blend everything in a liquidizer until smooth and
serve chilled in glasses, topped, if liked, with chopped
hazelnuts, brazils, cashews or flaked almonds.

Dried Fruit Compote

This dessert has to be planned several hours in
advance, as the dried fruit needs soaking beforehand.
It is a very easy dish to make, though. The quantities
given below need not be adhered to exactly, and you
can substitute other kinds of dried fruit if you wish.

8oz (225g) Hunza apricots
2oz (50g) dried prunes
2oz (50g) dried bananas
2oz (50g) dried figs
2oz (50g) dried apples
2oz (50g) raisins

1 pint (600ml) water
4 whole cloves
2 inch (5cm) stick cinnamon
1 tablespoon apple juice concentrate, or 1 teaspoon
organic honey

PREPARATION TIME: (excluding time for soaking
fruit) 15 minutes
COOKING TIME: 30 minutes

Soak the dried fruits overnight in the water with the
spices and apple juice concentrate or honey. The next
day, transfer to a saucepan and bring to the boil.
Reduce the heat and simmer for about 25 minutes.
Remove the spices before serving. This compote can be
served either hot or cold, on its own or covered with
crunchy topping (see page 311). If served hot, it goes
down well with low-fat yoghurt or nut cream (see
page 316).

No-Cook Cake

This uncooked cake tastes just as good as, if not better
than, standard baked cakes.

8oz (225g) oatflakes, fine, coarse or medium – it
doesn't matter
4oz (125g) cashews, brazils or almonds, ground

1 banana, mashed
1 carrot, grated
juice 1 lemon
1 dessertspoon organic honey
water or soya milk to mix
strawberries, raspberries or fresh apricots to garnish

PREPARATION TIME: 15 minutes
COOKING TIME: nil

In a large mixing bowl, combine all the ingredients except the fruit for garnish, adding just enough water or soya milk – or you could use ordinary skimmed milk – to make the mixture moist and sticky. Press into a shallow cake tin, decorate with fresh fruit and chill for 1–2 hours. Serve with yoghurt or nut cream (see below).

Nut Cream

All my life I have been a lover of double cream, clotted cream, top of the milk, tinned cream even. The thicker and gooier the better. That is, I was until I discovered nut cream – a healthier and really far nicer kind of cream. Now, I never buy dairy cream and hardly ever have it when eating out. Nut creams are nice, and definitely not naughty.

Although very few restaurants make nut creams yet, they are very easy to make at home and I have found them extremely popular with guests. Nut creams don't taste exactly like dairy creams, but have a delightful taste all of their own. The vanilla essence is not essential, but highly recommended. It must be the real thing, not synthetic.

> 4oz (125g) cashew nuts or almonds, ground
> 1 teaspoon natural vanilla extract
> ¼ pint (150ml) water
> ½ teaspoon organic honey

PREPARATION TIME: about 5 minutes
COOKING TIME: nil

Put all the ingredients in a liquidizer and blend on high speed until completely smooth. Nut creams taste better if chilled, so keep in the fridge until required.

Carob Cream

Carob, the cellulite watcher's alternative to chocolate, can be used in any recipe that calls for chocolate. I must point out though that as chocolate is such a favourite food, many people find the taste and texture of carob disappointing. I did at first, but now I've got used to the less sweet, more powdery taste and I prefer it. It took a long time, though.

Carob cream can be used instead of ordinary or nut creams, and is good for spooning over fresh fruit. It turns simple fresh fruit into a proper dessert.

2oz (50g) cashew nuts, ground
3 tablespoons carob flour
1 teaspoon natural vanilla essence
1 teaspoon organic honey
a little water

PREPARATION TIME: about 5 minutes
COOKING TIME: nil

Blend all the ingredients together on high speed in a liquidizer until completely smooth. The thickness of the cream will depend on how much water you add. It is best to start off with very little water – say 2 tablespoons – and add as required while the cream is blending.

READY-MADE DESSERTS

If you are an ice-cream lover, look out for dairy-free ice-creams. These are increasingly available and offer a delicious alternative to those made with either dairy ingredients or 'non-milk fat', whatever that may be. They do not taste exactly the same as dairy ice-cream but have a wonderful taste of their own. *Sweet Sensation* is a range of non-dairy, lactose-free frozen desserts.

Flavours include raspberry ripple, tutti-frutti, black cherry, and vanilla. *Maranelli's* also make an 'ice supreme' with organic soya milk, in chocolate, vanilla and raspberry flavours. These ices are sweetened with apple juice, not sugar.

Berrydale's make a non-dairy ice-cream in a range of flavours. The ingredients are tofu, honey, soya milk, apple concentrate and flavouring. These ices are also low in cholesterol and are lactose-free.

Plamil produces a range of soya desserts which do not have to be kept in the fridge.

Chapter 22

Packed Lunches and Eating Out

Although most canteens, school cafeterias and college refectories now serve vegetarian meals, it is still not all that easy to find the right sort of food when you are eating out. Often the only answer is to pack up your own lunch before leaving the house in the mornings.

This does not have to involve lengthy preparations. For example, you can spread hummous on oatcakes or barleycakes, cover with fresh alfalfa sprouts, cucumber or tomatoes, and season with pepper for a wonderful, healthy sandwich.

Any of the dips or spreads in the chapter on starters make very good sandwich spreads. You do not need butter or margarine. Sesame or sunflower seed spread is delicious in a sandwich, especially when tomatoes, lettuce or cucumber are added. You can also chop up into small pieces carrots, green, red and yellow peppers, and broccoli or cauliflower for crudités. You should not wrap sandwiches in tinfoil (aluminium, which we now know is very bad for us) but in cling-wrap or old-fashioned greaseproof paper instead.

Then add a low-fat yoghurt, an apple, banana or other fruit in season, and you have a perfect packed lunch. A tub of plain cottage cheese or a packet of quark will take care of your protein needs if you want a change from yoghurt.

Whenever possible, drink mineral or filtered water. Try not to buy fizzy drinks, even the low-calorie kind, as they contain all sorts of nasties. Aqua Libra is good but very expensive. Most fruit juices are really too concentrated for the cellulite-watcher so dilute them with mineral water whenever possible.

Most supermarkets now sell ready-prepared fresh salads. Marks and Spencer do a vast range, and although they may seem expensive they often work out cheaper than buying a whole cauliflower or a whole pound of broccoli, for instance, and then not being able to use it all up.

What if you are in a situation where you cannot avoid eating out? Well, obviously once in a while it does no harm to eat a cheese sandwich, an ice-cream composed entirely of artificial ingredients, or a take-away meal. However, as you proceed with the anti-cellulite diet, you become less and less able to eat junk food. It just tastes horrible, and makes you feel too full and uncomfortable. The more 'good' food you eat, the more refined your system becomes, and the less able to digest artificial or over-sugared or salted foods.

At the time of writing, food on trains is still in the dark ages. Even now, there is absolutely nothing I can eat in the dining car, and the 'great British breakfast' or the highly expensive 'Continental' version contains everything a cellulite-watcher should avoid. The buffet car is no better. Occasionally, there are some Granny Smith apples but otherwise – nothing. It is the same with buffet facilities in the stations – there is just nothing I can eat.

My solution is to pack up something suitable for myself before I travel, because I know for a fact that I will not be able to find anything I can eat either on the train or at the station.

Airports and airlines, by contrast, have improved out of all recognition in the past few years. When flying, I always order the vegan menu about twenty-four hours in advance, and it is usually absolutely delicious. It comes with herbal tea, and also you are served first, to the envy of the other passengers. The vegetarian menu available, so far as I know, on all airlines, is also consistently good in my experience. Most main airports have salad and health bars where you can buy exactly the sort of food you should be eating.

For many of us, eating out at an expensive restaurant is a treat. But expensive restaurants are geared more to gourmets than to providing truly nourishing food. Most high-priced restaurants rely on taste sensations, exotica, complicated sauces, expensive meats – none of which you need. However, I must say that in my years of being a strict vegetarian I have never experienced any real problem in restaurants. Usually there is a starter or two that is acceptable, and you can always ask for a plate of plain steamed vegetables, or a large salad. Wherever possible avoid steak bars and steak houses, as they often serve only peas or fried mushrooms as vegetables – they too are stuck in the dark ages over food, and imagine that meat has to dominate every plate while the rest of the food is merely a garnish to make the dish look pretty. As a general rule, the more expensive the restaurant, the more likely that they will be able to provide you with a plate of plain vegetables, or plainly cooked fish if you are not vegetarian.

Motorway menus are surprisingly good. A few years ago, motorway cafés were heavily criticized, but I have found that I can always get something suitable to eat at them. Most have extensive salad ranges, and chains like Little Chef have introduced a very acceptable range of vegetarian dishes. Motorway cafés all sell mineral water now, and most have herbal teas as well. When I have to travel long distances on motorways I never worry about getting something suitable to eat en route.

What about dinner parties? Again, it does no harm to indulge in cream sauces or Black Forest gâteau once in a while, but there is really no need, as I see it, to eat food that you don't like or shouldn't be having just because you are a guest in somebody else's house. Very often, older people do not understand vegetarian or healthy cooking.

In these situations I occasionally say to the people concerned that I wouldn't want them to go to all the fuss and worry of trying to prepare something suitable, so if they don't mind I will bring my own food. This practice is increasingly accepted nowadays, as many people are on unusual diets and cannot always expect their host or hostess to prepare something special.

I do not go along with the view that you must eat gratefully what your host or hostess has prepared. If the food does not agree with me then I don't eat it. At parties, receptions, weddings, and other such occasions I have frequently been unable to eat any of the food at all.

The answer is to prepare for this eventuality. If I am going to an occasion where I cannot be sure that there will be something suitable for me to eat, I take something to keep me going – an apple or two, a banana, some nuts, an unsweetened carob bar. You can soon get into the habit of doing this.

Alcoholic drinks are not allowed on the anti-cellulite diet. This is partly because they contain large amounts of sugar in the form of empty calories. But the other, more important aspect is that the body treats alcohol as a poison and starts to attempt to detoxify it as soon as it enters the bloodstream. This means that alcohol adds to the toxic load on the liver, which at its best can detoxify only one unit – that's one glass of sherry, half a pint of lager or a single measure of spirits

– in an hour. So if you drink faster than this, excess alcohol will stay in the bloodstream. If it is not detoxified, it will turn to fat and eventually, to cellulite. So it is best avoided, at least on a daily basis.

You should never drink extra-strong lagers, which contain huge amounts of sugar, and ideally you should avoid lager altogether, as well as spirits and fortified wines such as port or sherry. Your system can cope with an occasional glass of champagne or wine, especially if it is organic. In fact, whenever buying wines look for organic labels. These are becoming widely available in supermarkets and wine shops. When drinking champagne, intersperse it with non-fizzy mineral water. If you drink the sparkling kind, you will accumulate too much gas and bloating will result.

Eating out just takes a little thought, a little adjustment – and then it becomes an automatic part of your life.

Bibliography

Campion, Kitty: *A Woman's Herbal*, Century, 1987

Davies, Dr Stephen and Stewart, Dr Alan: *Nutritional Medicine*, Pan, 1987

Davis, Patricia: *Aromatherapy: An A–Z*, C. W. Daniel, 1988

Gray, Dr Robert: *The Colon Health Handbook*, Rockridge Publishing Company, California, 1983

Hepper, Camilla: *Herbal Cosmetics*, Thorsons, 1987

Kenton, Leslie: *The Joy of Beauty*, Century, 1983

Kenton, Leslie and Kenton, Susannah: *Raw Energy Recipes*, Century, 1985

Maxwell-Hudson, Clare: *The Complete Book of Massage*, Dorling Kindersley, 1988

Maxwell-Hudson, Clare: *Your Health and Beauty Book*, Macdonald, 1979

Maxwell-Hudson, Clare: *The Natural Beauty Book*, Macdonald, 1983

Ryman, Danièle: *The Aromatherapy Handbook*, Century, 1984

Soltanoff, Dr Jack: *Natural Healing*, Warner Books (USA), 1988

Tisserand, Robert: *The Art of Aromatherapy*, C. W. Daniel, 1977

Tisserand, Robert: *Aromatherapy for Everyone*, Penguin, 1988

Valnet, Dr Jean: *The Practice of Aromatherapy*, C. W. Daniel, 1982

West, Ouida: *The Magic of Massage*, Century, 1983

Wright, Brian: *Cleansing the Colon*, Green Press, 1987

Wright, Celia: *The Wright Diet*, Piatkus, 1986

Useful Addresses

Aromatherapy courses

The London School of
  Aromatherapy,
PO Box 780
London NW6 5EQ

Also has a list of trained
aromatherapists in the
UK and other parts of the
world. Principal: Patricia
Davis.

The International
  Federation of
  Aromatherapists
46 Dalkeith Road
Dulwich
London SE21 8LS

This organization has a
list of accredited schools
and colleges, as well as
individual
aromatherapists. It is a
registered charity.

Aromatherapy Oils
(mail order)

Bodytreats Ltd
15 Approach Road
Raynes Park
London SW20 8BA

Micheline Arcier
  Aromatherapy
7 William Street
London SW1

Neal's Yard Apothecary
Neal's Yard
Covent Garden
London WC2

The Nutri Centre
7 Park Crescent
London W1N 3HE
0171 436 5122

Body brushes

Higher Nature
Burwash Common
East Sussex TN19 7LA
01435 882880

Kitty Campion
The Natural Health and
    Iridology Centre
19 Park Terrace
Tunstall
Stoke-on-Trent
Staffs ST6 6PB
Kitty will also help with
anti-cellulite treatments.

Nutri Centre, as above.

Sources of Help

Sally Gilbert Wilson
56 Harley Street
London NW1 5HW

Nutritional Information

For advice on detoxifying
and cleansing diets,
contact the sources listed
above, or:

The Nutritional Advisory
    Service
PO Box 268
Hove,
East Sussex BN3 1R3

Massage Courses

The Claire Maxwell-
    Hudson School of
    Massage
PO Box 457
London NW2 4BR

Note: please enclose large
s.a.e. when writing to any
of these addresses.

Index